'A book of dignity, sincerity, and breathtaking beauty ...
David Servan-Schreiber helps us look at death and prepare
ourselves to die *well*. It's a very powerful read that
inspires deep appreciation' *Le Point*

'A book that is as lucid as it is personal. This little book
may be where the psychiatrist takes his leave [and] in his
own manner: brave, bright, committed' *Le Temps*

'A very personal account, intense and moving,
simple and sincere' *Psychologies*

'A poignant final book about the return of cancer.
This is also a time for David Servan-Schreiber to say
goodbye to those who have loved his books'
Le Monde, 'Book of the Day'

'[Servan-Schreiber] talks about women and love, his
children, his companions in misfortune... and about the
importance of giving meaning to life so that we can depart
in peace. Such a lesson in courage inspires us to live
our own lives to the fullest' *Gala*

'David Servan-Schreiber shows true empathy and emotion.
His sincerity and honesty also deeply touch the reader'
Livres Hebdo

'The courageous testimony he delivers, with the urgency of
an end he knows is imminent, is a life lesson addressed to his
readers and patients, his family, and perhaps also to doctors'
Le Quotidien du médecin

'An intimate, moving little book that is full of hope'
L'Est Républicain

Also by David Servan-Schreiber

Healing Without Freud or Prozac
Anticancer

not the
last goodbye

reflections on
life, death, healing and cancer

dr david servan-schreiber

with ursula gauthier

MACMILLAN

First published 2011 by Editions Robert Laffont

First published in Great Britain 2011 by Macmillan
an imprint of Pan Macmillan, a division of Macmillan Publishers Limited
Pan Macmillan, 20 New Wharf Road, London N1 9RR
Basingstoke and Oxford
Associated companies throughout the world
www.panmacmillan.com

ISBN 978-0-230-76372-2

9 8 7 6 5 4 3 2 1

A CIP catalogue record for this book is available from the British Library.

Typeset by seagulls.net
Printed by CPI Group (UK) Ltd. Croydon, CR0 4YY

Visit **www.panmacmillan.com** to read more about all our books and to
buy them. You will also find features, author interviews and news of any
author events, and you can sign up for e-newsletters so that you're always
first to hear about our new releases.

This book is dedicated to the cancer specialists who have so generously given me their time, expertise and support ever since my cancer was discovered, by sheer accident, nineteen years ago.

It is also dedicated to all my patients who have endured similar ordeals. They have inspired in me courage, determination and inner strength.

Finally, I dedicate this book to my three children: sixteen-year-old Sacha, two-year-old Charlie, and Anna, who is six months old. It would grieve me deeply if I were unable to accompany them in their journey through life. I hope that I have contributed to their vital life-force and that they will know to nourish it in their hearts, so that it can spring to their aid whenever they are faced with life's challenges.

May 2011

part I

1

the bike test

That day, when I left the radiology clinic, I decided to ride my bike home. I have always loved to cycle around Paris, and I remember that ride as a special moment. Of course, after the news I'd just received, it would have been wiser to take a taxi, as the city's uneven cobblestones were dangerous for someone in my condition. But it was precisely because of the news I'd been given that I needed some fresh air.

It was 16 June 2010. I had just undergone an MRI and the results were far from encouraging. The images showed a gigantic, vein-filled mass occupying the cavity in my frontal lobe, the site of two previous operations many years earlier. My oncologist was hesitant. He didn't believe the tumour had returned; it was more likely a large oedema, a delayed reaction to my previous bouts of radiotherapy. But he wasn't sure. We needed to wait for the opinion of a radiologist who was away and wouldn't be back for several days.

Tumour or oedema, either way this thing that was flourishing in my frontal lobe was a direct threat to my life. Given its size and the pressure it was exerting inside my cranium, the slightest variation in internal pressure – a bump or jolt – could kill me or leave me severely disabled. And I'd just returned from a three-day trip to the United States, with this ticking bomb inside my head. Each pocket of turbulence could have been the end of me.

Leaving the radiology clinic, I called my wife. 'It's not looking good,' I told her, and burst into tears. I could hear her sobbing on the other end of the line. I was devastated. With such a weight on my shoulders I couldn't bring myself to cross town cooped up in a car. Instead I got on my bike, fully aware of the risk I was about to take.

When I tell my friends this story, they look at me in astonishment. The David they know is neither desperate nor easily discouraged. So why would I act so carelessly? Was it a fleeting suicidal impulse? A romantic wish to die on the cobbled streets of Paris? An attempt to escape the months of pain and anxiety that surely lay ahead of me?

Usually I respond with a quip: 'But I couldn't possibly leave my bike there! I love it too much – it's my Tornado. It would be like Zorro abandoning his faithful steed in the wilderness!' The truth is, despite what my oncologist said, and no matter how much I wanted to believe him, I feared the worst. I had my back to the wall.

I felt a sudden urge to test my courage. To see whether, in this decisive battle, I would be able to mobilize as much strength as I'd found for my two previous operations. With twenty more years on the clock and a far larger tumour – if that's what it was – in my head, I was going to need every ounce of courage and composure I could muster.

As crazy and reckless as it might seem, the 'bike test' did the trick: cycling home was a reminder that no matter what the diagnosis, my desire to live was very much intact, as was my determination. I knew I wouldn't give up.

2

exhaustion

The first signs that something was wrong had appeared in May 2010, about six weeks before the MRI. On a few occasions, my legs simply gave way, as if all the strength had been suddenly sucked out of them. I clearly remember standing in my office looking for a book on the shelf one moment, and the next I was on my knees on the floor, without the slightest warning.

A few days later, I was being interviewed for French television about Bernard Giraudeau. Bernard was a French actor and film director who had become a friend during his battle with cancer. The journalist informed me that Bernard wasn't doing well. I was distraught at the news and found the interview very difficult. When it was over I stood up to show the journalist out. Just as I was saying goodbye, I collapsed, taking her down with me. The video camera toppled onto me, the coffee table tipped over, covering the floor with tea, cups and everything else that had been on top. The journalist called for help, bringing the whole office rushing over to where I lay slumped on the floor. It was pretty embarrassing. The journalist couldn't hide her concern. I could just imagine her thinking, 'Oh my God, another Bernard Giraudeau!' I tried to reassure her. 'I've just got back from the United States, and I'm jetlagged. I've also been having dizzy spells lately. But don't worry; I'm taking care of it.'

These symptoms didn't really tally with a neurological problem, or with a recurrence of my tumour. None of the alarm bells associated with cancer were ringing. My last scan in January had been perfectly clean and the next one was scheduled for July. After considering a number of possible explanations, I concluded that my frailty must be due to anaemia. I had been taking a lot of ibuprofen for back pain, and thought that perhaps the medication had caused an ulcer in my digestive tract, which was bleeding and thereby bringing on both the anaemia and the vertigo. I promised myself I would go for a check-up as soon as possible.

At the time, I was constantly on the go; following the publication of my book *Anticancer,* I was taking part in conferences and appearing on radio and TV, especially in the United States, where the book was generating widespread interest. So I put my fatigue down to repeated air travel, jetlag and the stress of public speaking.

Shortly after the French TV interview where I'd collapsed, despite feeling unwell, I had to make a quick transatlantic trip to Detroit for an important public television programme. When I arrived at the studio, I was as white as a sheet. 'You're going to have to work wonders,' I told the make-up artist. 'Don't worry,' she replied in a midwestern drawl. 'We'll make you look just spiffy!' During the following two hours on set, I gave it my best: I smiled, I was upbeat, and I did indeed look spiffy. Afterwards, however, I was completely drained and went straight back to my hotel. I had a plane to catch the next morning and wanted to get as much sleep as possible.

Waking up the next morning was an even taller order. I had a splitting headache, and it took all of my strength to get out of bed and force down some breakfast. On the way to the airport, I had to pull over at a pharmacy to pick up some Tylenol. Searching through the aisles, I collapsed with a crash into a shelf, knocking its contents to the floor. People in the shop helped me to my feet and insisted I go to the hospital. Not wanting to miss my flight to Paris, I got back into the taxi instead.

But I could no longer deny that something was wrong. From the car I called a friend in Paris, and asked him to schedule an emergency MRI for me. I also called my mother, who I knew would be available, and asked her to pick me up when I arrived. My legs felt so unsteady that I was afraid I wouldn't be able to make it home on my own. And sure enough, I fell several times at the airport in Detroit.

3

the big one

I had the MRI the day after my return from Detroit. When I grasped the magnitude of this thing that had been growing in my brain over the past four months, I made a conscious decision then and there not to look at the scans. I preferred, and I still prefer, not to put negative images in my head, even if my oncologist continued to insist that it wasn't a tumour. To this day I still haven't seen them. I wasn't being superstitious, but I believe in the effect images can have on both body and mind. I'm convinced that we shouldn't look at things that frighten us too much; fear, as we all know, gives poor counsel. Later, when I learned that this so-called oedema was in fact a malignant tumour, I found out as much as I could about it in order better to defend myself. But I did not want to 'pollute' myself with images which were so intimidating that they might shake my confidence, might make me think: 'This time, I won't make it.'

In a way I was in denial. But studies have shown that denial is not always a bad defence mechanism, particularly in situations where the prognosis is very poor or the odds are unfavourable. There are two types of denial. The first is seen in patients who are so terrified by their illness that they would rather blind themselves to it, to the extent that they might not even seek treatment. This is an extremely dangerous attitude. The second type of denial is well known to all those who, on the contrary, take care of their health and follow the guidance of their doctors. These are the people who know that a positive state of mind helps you to live well, and can even help you to heal. I have thought a lot about this, and I believe that anything that enhances life also strengthens the life-force within us. Likewise, anything that erodes our desire to live also diminishes our capacity to heal.

After all, an oedema was more reassuring. Of course, a little voice inside my head kept whispering, 'Too good to be true.' While I waited to hear the radiologist's opinion, I decided to travel to Le Mans in western France, where I was scheduled to give a talk to two hundred journalists at an international conference on the theme of fighting fatigue. Given my own state of exhaustion, this was not without its irony, but I didn't want to cancel at the last minute.

I was in my hotel room the night before the event when I collapsed on my way to the bathroom and had to drag myself over to the bed. The next morning, I was feeling better. But as I climbed out of my cab, I fell over again.

What's more, my vision was out of focus and my eyes had developed quite a pronounced squint. For a moment I actually thought about giving my lecture with sunglasses on. In the end, I addressed the problem by sweeping my gaze from right to left across the auditorium while I spoke. No one seemed to notice that my eyes were looking in different directions.

The following day I was due to go to Cologne for a long-scheduled work meeting. As I was still so unsteady on my feet, my brother Emile decided to take the train with me. Leaving the station in Cologne, I keeled over again. Emile insisted that I go to A&E. I recalled the brilliant neurosurgeons I'd met a few months earlier at the University Hospital of Cologne during a three-day training seminar I had led on the themes of *Anticancer*. I had been impressed by their open-mindedness and their use of ultra-specialized techniques. We telephoned one of the neurosurgeons with whom I had got along well. When I described my symptoms and the results of the MRI, she could not have been clearer: 'Take a taxi,' she said. 'Come right away.' It wasn't exactly reassuring, but at the same time I knew I was in good hands. I immediately had an emergency MRI. This time the diagnosis was unquestionable: it wasn't an oedema – it was a relapse.

And not just any relapse. It was *the* relapse. The nasty, quasi-final one. 'The Big One', as Californians call the terrible earthquake that may one day hit the West Coast. I knew the prognosis. Sooner or later, it would come back. I could slow down the inevitable; I could gain a few years. But there was nothing I could do to make this cancer disappear for ever. So this was it. The thing I'd been dreading all these years had finally happened.

To be completely honest, a part of me had started to believe, secretly, that the cancer wouldn't return. But my more rational side had never stopped reminding me that it would. I told myself, 'I'll cross that bridge when I come to it.'

And that's what I did. Just as my 'bike test' had encouraged me to hope, I still had some fight left in me.

4

bedridden
in cologne

The tumour was so large, and it was pressing down on my brain to such an extent, that the Cologne doctors decided that I should undergo surgery immediately.

I was extremely lucky in my bad fortune. If there was one hospital where I would have wanted to be operated on, this was it. The University Hospital of Cologne embraces a rare, and in my eyes invaluable, philosophy: while championing the use of cutting-edge technology, it is also open to alternative methods. What's more, it is willing to combine them. The Department of Complementary and Alternative Medicine conducts joint research projects with the Department of Neurosurgery on innovative therapeutic methods that combine the two approaches, and their findings are published in the most prestigious cancer journals in the world.

During the training seminar I had led at the university, I'd been very impressed by the revolutionary methods that were being developed by neurosurgeons there. One in particular involves implanting tiny radioactive beads – after the surgical removal of the tumour – into the brain in the exact location affected by the cancer. The action of these beads is concentrated and highly localized, destroying cancerous cells that might have remained after the surgery. This new technique is infinitely more precise than traditional external radiation therapy, where the wide radioactive beams attack both the tumour and the healthy tissue surrounding it. It also has far fewer side effects. The Cologne neurosurgeons assured me: 'We have very good success rates with this method. If your tumour should return, remember that we can help you.'

I was too sick to travel and could return to France only if I was repatriated by an official medical team. Nevertheless I was reluctant to have an operation in Cologne, so far from home. Thankfully everyone at the hospital was very caring. Some of the doctors and nurses spoke excellent French and they were delighted to practise it with me.

My brothers and my friends sometimes ask me whether I was ever discouraged, that summer, by the relentless nature of the illness – the need for yet another operation, another bout of radiation, maybe even more chemotherapy. Did I, even fleetingly, feel like giving up? I answer without hesitation: 'Never.' It's not because I'm particularly heroic. I think people tend to get discouraged when the suffering has been going on too long. The nausea, the disability, the humiliation, these are all forms of suffering. So far, I've been spared these trials for the most part. I hope it will last.

I knew straight away, without a shadow of a doubt, I was going to do whatever it took to fight this cancer. I was going to find the conventional therapies best adapted to tackling my condition, and I would back them up with my anticancer programme. Of course, with my strength diminished, I would have to restrict my physical exercise. Cycling, for example, had become too dangerous. A tumour of this size, particularly in the frontal lobe, greatly increases the risk of epilepsy, and you're better off having a seizure on foot than on a bicycle. Still, there was nothing to stop me from walking, and I was determined to walk for at least half an hour each day. At the same time, I would continue to fight the tumour on every other front: through nutrition, yoga and meditation.

5

the land of the living

My brothers Franklin and Edouard quickly joined Emile at my bedside. Their presence was vital for me. I was so exhausted that I couldn't think clearly or make decisions. There was a mountain of logistical tasks to accomplish: the hospital admission formalities, of course, but also discussions with the doctors about what the surgery would entail, how I would need to prepare for it, and who would be there to help me during my hospitalization. Maybe it was the pressure of the tumour on my brain, but I felt my mind failing me. I needed the support of people I could completely trust.

My wife, who was pregnant at the time, couldn't come to Cologne as often as she would have liked. Moreover, because my operation would be followed by the implantation of radioactive beads, I would be emitting radiation that could be harmful to the baby. To console us through this forced separation, we kept in contact with long, tender phone conversations that greatly comforted me.

The support of my loved ones was like a gift from heaven. I am enormously lucky to belong to a large family – four brothers and about twenty cousins, joined together by a powerful bond. They pulled out all the stops to come to my aid at this critical time. While I was in the hospital in Cologne, my brothers took turns visiting me so that I was never alone. Each night one of them slept on a bed close to me. I remember the night when I got up to go to the bathroom and woke up the brother who was with me... by falling over him. Once we'd got over the shock, we had a good laugh about it.

Although the operation was a very serious one, we ended up spending some wonderful moments together. In the morning we listened to music, at night we watched movies. During the day we would admire the pretty German nurses going about their work (a restorative activity I can highly recommend). My stay in the hospital coincided with the football World Cup, which I watched avidly. At last I was able to indulge in an interest that I had neglected for years because of the demands of my work.

The hospital food, on the other hand, was a problem. My meals often consisted of slices of salami and processed cheese on white bread – more or less the polar opposite of an anticancer diet. Thankfully, my mother had struck up a friendship with the owner of Bella Vista, an excellent local Italian restaurant, and they spoiled me with delicious Mediterranean dishes that they prepared specially.

Sacha, my fifteen-year-old son, came to visit me too. He lives in the United States with his mother, so we don't see each other often. We had of course spoken every day on the phone, and I could sense he was very anxious – not only for my health, but also, less openly, because he feared that the disease might have changed me. On his first night in Cologne, we spent several hours together. He was sharing a room with my mother, and afterwards he touchingly confided in her, 'You know, I feel a lot better now, because he's still my dad. He hasn't changed.'

When I was in the convalescent home after my surgery, my brothers organized a 'rota' for the people who came to visit me and sometimes even spent the night in a spare room in the centre. This was no small task, as a great many friends came to see me during my two months in Cologne.

Anyone who has had a serious illness understands how lonely the experience can be. You can't turn over in your sleep by yourself, can't sit down in a chair without help, can't make phone calls or answer emails. Disability doesn't just make daily life difficult; it can also strip you of your dignity. While I was in the hospital, I was convinced that I smelled awful, even though, with great kindness, the nurses helped me wash every day. All I wanted was to be able to take a shower before they arrived, to spare them from having to deal with a patient who didn't smell like a bed of roses. But when all's said and done, having an entourage of friends and family is an extraordinary blessing. For a patient, it makes all the difference to be able to count on help to have a shower, to brush your teeth, to eat, get dressed, get up or go to bed.

The emotional dimension is important too. The sicker you are, the lonelier you feel, and the more anxious and depressed you become. Whereas the more you are surrounded by loved ones, the more you remain connected to life and to everything that makes you want to live. It doesn't take much: watching a movie together, playing cards, telling each other stories and evoking memories, planning weekends and holidays. Even if sometimes you have to give up your lifestyle from 'before', as a patient you need to feel that you're still part of the club – the club of the living, of people who do things and get on with their lives.

6

back in the fish tank

My previous experiences of being hospitalized had taught me that the beginning of the treatment phase is fairly plain sailing. You no longer have to worry about what will happen the next day, or even in the next hour. Instead, you wage innumerable tiny battles. You get up, you eat, you try to stay as comfortable as possible despite the head aches, the nausea, the injections and all the other phys ical pain. You find the strength to speak, to listen, to stay connected. These are minor battles, but as they follow on relentlessly one after another, they demand all your attention. And then there are the more important battles: the medical tests, the anaesthesia, the operation. You devote whatever strength you have left to the most essential thing of all: safeguarding your relationship with your family, your children, your siblings...

For days after the operation I suffered a terrible headache, a shooting pain that was worse than anything I'd known before, which was not surprising given the size of the tumour that had just been removed. The pain was inescapable. I couldn't read or eat or watch television. I couldn't do anything. Fortunately hospitals are now good at tackling this sort of pain and I ended up asking for morphine, which can be administered nowadays without creating dependency.

Of all of the trials you have to endure while in hospital, the one I fear the most is anaesthesia. It means an injection, and I don't like needles, even though (or perhaps because) I've had to submit to so many. Above all, you lose control over your thoughts. One moment you are there, and the next – *pff* – nothing. This sensation of total disconnection is even more terrifying when the operation involves the brain. Woody Allen famously once said, 'My brain? That's my second-favourite organ.' But for me it comes first. I love the mind. I've given a lot of my life to it, I've trained it, I've prepared it for certain tasks. The idea that someone is going to remove a large part of it is very alarming.

I remember, twenty years ago, how afraid I was the first time I had to undergo brain surgery. I knew the surgeons would cut as widely as possible around the tumour so as not to miss any malignant cells. As soon as I emerged from the anaesthetic, the first thing I did was to drum out some 'scales' on the bedsheets with my left hand, to check that they hadn't taken away too many important things from my right lobe. I felt enormous relief when my fingers obeyed me.

In addition to the motor skills, when you intervene in the frontal lobe you also run the more disturbing risk of creating psychological, in particular emotional, changes. I wanted to continue to love what I loved and to feel the same emotions I'd always had. I wanted to continue to hate, admire or despise the same things I'd always hated, admired or despised. Before my first operation, I was terrified that I might wake up with a different personality from the one I had gone to sleep with. Would I recognize myself when I regained consciousness or would there be a stranger living in my brain? Or would I gradually discover that I wasn't the same person? After how long? And suppose I *did* recognize myself when I woke up – how could I be sure I was really me?

My brothers, who were already standing by me back then, were my rocks in this storm. They calmed me. They reassured me that I hadn't changed much. The most that they had noticed was that I had perhaps become more emotional than before. I was more prone to cry, during a sentimental movie, for example, or while listening to music. When I recovered, I returned to my work as a psychiatrist, and I noticed that I was far more sensitive than before. This was in fact a significant change, above all in my professional life. I discovered, with wonder, that my patients had the ability to touch me deeply.

Swapping places, experiencing the worries, suffering and hopes of a patient, helped me become more human, more receptive to our common condition. But I'm convinced that in my case the surgery played an important role because I became particularly sensitive, even excessively so, as if I could no longer distance myself from my emotions.

So the operation last summer was the third time someone went into my brain. For the third time I ran the risk of losing my soul. It was with real dread that I thought about the anaesthetic. Thankfully, when I woke up, as on the previous occasions I felt that I was more or less the same person. I was groggy but very relieved to come back to myself, and to encounter the same thoughts swimming around in the familiar fish tank of my mind.

7

the vampire
of leuven

A week later, the time came to implant the radioactive beads that would 'clean up' any residual cancer cells which had infiltrated tissue the scalpel hadn't reached. These beads would automatically emit radiation until they expired. The effect, as with external radiation therapy, would not be immediately measurable.

I wanted to add another innovative approach to my treatment, one that is still in the experimental stage: a made-to-measure 'vaccine' concocted for my own tumour. The Pittsburgh hospital where I worked for many years has one of a handful of programmes around the world that are testing this fascinating new method; it has already shown its impact on cancers, including brain cancer. But it was out of the question for me to travel across the Atlantic. By a stroke of luck, my brother Franklin discovered that a patient had benefited from a similar treatment in Leuven in Belgium, just 110 miles away from where I was.

We learned that the team directed by Professor Stefaan Van Gool at the University of Leuven was at the forefront of the field, having treated 170 cases. Moreover, my case fitted nicely into their research protocol.

The method practised in Leuven involves removing 20 per cent of the patient's white blood cells and then, in the lab, bringing them into contact with the tumour that has been extracted by surgery, thus sensitizing the blood cells to the proteins that are present on the surface of the tumour cells. Then, these 'conditioned' white blood cells are re-injected periodically into the patient, and act in his or her body exactly as a vaccine would: they alert the immune system to any element that possesses these particular proteins on its surface. The little soldiers of the immune system can thus track down the cancer cells in every nook and cranny of the patient's organism, wherever they might be hiding.

No other technique has such a targeted approach. Compared with these 'hyper-surgical strikes', chemotherapy looks like a napalm attack, or carpet-bombing. And the method has had very good results. According to current statistics, the vaccine manages to totally clean up 20 per cent of tumours. A complete cure for one in five cancers – that's a very impressive score.

This ground-breaking concept, which essentially informs the immune system so that it can mobilize one hundred per cent against a clearly labelled enemy, is currently being used to fight certain brain cancers, melanomas, kidney cancers and cervical cancer. In the future, increasing numbers of patients will be able to benefit from this approach.

Shortly after my surgery, Franklin took me to the University of Leuven where 20 per cent of my white blood cells were removed. A metal syringe was inserted into the crook of my elbow to extract my blood so that it could then be circulated outside my body five times via a centrifuge, which would separate out the white blood cells. I couldn't help thinking of this machine as a kind of vampire while it sucked out my blood on one side and re-injected it on the other. The process was also very long.

After two hours, when the needle in my arm had really begun to throb, I asked the nurses, 'Will it take much longer?' They replied, 'It's almost over, only two and a half hours left.' And I only had an audio book to help me through, and not the most uplifting one either: *David Copperfield*.

The experience was so gruelling that when I had to do it again – for a second batch of the vaccine – I came prepared. I brought two movies: a charming animated film that I highly recommend: *Spirit, Stallion of the Cimarron*, and the hilarious *Mrs Doubtfire*. As soon as I got there, I summoned my courage and pleaded, 'Please, can you not put the needle in my arm this time? It hurts too much.' The reaction of the medical team surprised me: they weren't cross or annoyed; on the contrary, they were kind and understanding. They figured out another method, inserting a catheter in my neck, which was painless. It was a huge relief.

This incident taught me an important lesson: you shouldn't try to act like a hero in a hospital. As a doctor, I had a tendency to say, 'No problem, go ahead, stick the needle in,' even though I suffered as much as anyone else. I was approaching fifty, and it had taken me all those years to realize that you're better off being humble – and avoiding suffering.

8

cold shower

After major surgery, you know you're on the road to recovery when your appetite returns. You're hungry again, you crave certain foods or flavours. I have fond memories of the lunches I had in little bistros near the hospital. Sitting in the sun, with a marvellous plate of pasta and seafood, I could feel the joy of life flooding back to me. But the most overwhelming sign of recovery is the return of another appetite: desire. The first time I made love to my wife after my surgery, I felt I had become a man again. Desire and tenderness, both at once: that's the beauty of sex. Even if a hospital room that can't be locked from the inside is hardly the ideal place for a romantic reunion...

When I returned to Paris, I went back to a more or less normal life. I couldn't ride my bike any more, or go to the office, and I had to rest and take daily naps. Still, my legs grew stronger, my left eye was realigning itself, my squint was fading and I could read again. I began working from home, answering my emails, giving interviews by phone. I even managed to give a lecture on alternative medicine organized by the Association of Surgeons of the Netherlands. On the face of it, this academy wasn't the most receptive audience to this kind of approach, and I wasn't exactly on my best form. But I felt that I succeeded in sparking the interest of my listeners. I was on the right track, and was resolved to trust in the vaccine.

The first MRI check-up, in October, didn't reveal any suspicious shadows, and I had no physical symptoms – none of the migraines or rubbery legs of the previous spring. But the second MRI, in December, was a slap in the face. The tumour – well, actually, *a* tumour – was back. My wife, Gwenaëlle, who was eight months pregnant, had accompanied me to the radiology clinic. She was with me when they gave me the results. Her pain was indescribable. We were both so shell-shocked that we had to sit for a moment in the waiting room. Then we went and had lunch at a restaurant close to the hospital. We kept saying to each other, 'This is it. Here we go again,' and crying into our food. 'We'll do everything it takes,' Gwenaëlle said, 'like we always have. We're going to beat this. I'll be right here with you.'

In circumstances like these, the best antidote to despair is to focus on getting things done. But first you need to recognize that the situation is emotionally very difficult. You need to remind yourself that you'll be in this boat with your spouse, your family, your close friends. Only then can you confront the practical decisions and really commit yourself to action.

The tumour had grown back in the same place in my brain, but fortunately this time it was much smaller and less aggressive. It was probably a mutation of its predecessor, which might explain why the vaccine hadn't worked. The doctors told me, 'It's a perfect candidate for surgery, we can operate again right away.' I didn't have time to allow myself to become discouraged. I was operated on a week later.

This time the surgeons extracted the tumour entirely. The operation was so successful that no additional radiation was deemed necessary, and I was allowed to leave the hospital shortly afterwards. I decided not to go to a convalescent home to recuperate. My wife was due and it was very important for me to be present for the birth of my daughter, Anna. I wanted to be part of that magical experience, no matter what.

As for the vaccine, we had to start again from scratch. As the new tumour was a mutation, we needed to manufacture a new vaccine to try to fight it. The first attempt hadn't succeeded, but it was still a good idea. I hadn't forgotten the statistics: a 20 per cent success rate. It was worth a second try.

9

turning fifty: the elephant, the skull and the wind

The vaccine wasn't enough to stop the cancer. At the end of February, following the first four injections, a routine MRI showed what radiologists call 'areas of contrast'. In plain English, this means areas where cancer cells are present. Within a week, the symptoms appeared: persistent headaches, a dragging left leg, a recalcitrant left hand. The doctors concluded that the cancer was again progressing, and that in addition an oedema was compressing the cortex zone responsible for motor coordination. This time the neurosurgeons couldn't operate: there was no clearly delimited tumour, only diffuse cancer cells. It would be impossible for a scalpel to pick out the cells one by one.

In Leuven, they told me that the vaccine was probably at least partially responsible for the inability of the cells to form a tumour. It was probably contributing to maintaining sufficient immune pressure to stave off the proliferation. In the meantime, the malignant cells had infiltrated areas of my right motor cortex, compromising my ability to move my left leg and arm. With the help of my doctor, whom I trusted completely, I decided that my best option was an anti-angiogenic drug, Avastin, alongside the vaccine injections.

For the past few weeks I've been unable to type with both hands on a keyboard, and I've been having a lot of difficulty walking. I'm often tired. Reading has become a struggle. And I'm losing my voice, so I speak very softly, as if I were whispering in someone's ear. I'm pacing myself, conscious that I'll need all my strength to pull through.

This is the year I turned fifty. I gave a party, with the help of my brothers, on an evening in April that was filled with the soft warmth of a Paris spring. I invited everyone I love. Some of my friends were aware of my condition; others less so. I wanted to be the one to tell them the news, in my own words. I thought a great deal about the little speech I planned to give. Should I dot all the *i*s and cross all the *t*s, quote technical terms and statistics? Or was it better to stay vague?

I chose honesty. I couldn't hide the signs of my illness: my whispering voice, my weakened left leg and arm. More importantly, this might be the last birthday I would share with my friends and I wanted to speak with an open heart.

When there's an elephant in the room there's no point pretending you don't see it: you should talk about it, and call it by its name.

So that night I called the elephant by its name. I gave all the details. And I'll give them again now, to you my readers, who have done me the honour of appreciating my work and given me so much joy.

Since the relapse of my cancer in June 2010, I've undergone three operations, one bout of radiation, two vaccine protocols and an anti-angiogenic treatment. The tumour has returned in a much more aggressive form than the one I lived with for eighteen years. It's a stage-four glioblastoma, whose prognosis is among the worst of any type of cancer: a mean survival time of fifteen months. In other words, half the people who have this kind of tumour live less than fifteen months after their diagnosis, and the other half live more than fifteen months. In the case of a relapse, there's almost no chance of surviving more than eighteen months.

I then described my battle plan for stacking all the odds in my favour, drawing on both the support of some exceptional physicians and the complementary action of the anticancer programme.

It's possible I'll never celebrate my fifty-first birthday, but I'm glad to have been able to share some of the values that I care deeply about. These values are best described by the term *empowerment:* that vital ability to seize power over yourself and your destiny. Though there's still some way to go, I'm very proud that I have been able to contribute to the advancement of this concept in my own field, medicine.

There's a lovely image in the novel *Friday* by the French novelist Michel Tournier. Tournier describes a buffalo's skull hanging from a tree. Music escapes from it when the wind blows through it. The question is: who makes that music? Is it the skull, is it the wind, or is it the coming together of the two?

Creativity is a similar phenomenon. All of us during our lives and experiences are like that buffalo skull – with life blowing through, producing a unique melody. What a feeling of jubilation to discover that you don't have to be an artist to live a creative life!

The most important thing I've learned in the past twenty years of my career as a scientist is also the greatest discovery of modern ecology. It's the simple yet fundamental idea that life is the expression of relationships within a network; it is not a series of separate goals pursued by distinct individuals. This is as true of ants, giraffes and wolves as it is of humans. It's through my interactions with all the pioneers of human ecology that I have been lucky enough to express my own creativity and contribute to the community. I am extremely grateful for that.

part II

10

much ado
about nothing...

I was slowly emerging from the fog. Three days after my operation in June, my friend the writer Régis Debray came to visit me as he was passing through Cologne. He sat down beside my bed and said to me in a jovial voice, 'So, I guess raspberries and broccoli aren't enough.'

Something tells me that anyone picking up this book is probably asking themselves the same question. The author of *Anticancer* suffers a serious relapse and is perhaps dying, or could even (I can't exclude the possibility) be dead as you read these words. All that, for this? The thousands of scientific articles pored over and analysed in detail; all that research dissected; those results cross-checked and weighed; the entire anticancer programme carefully adjusted, updated and altered to reflect new findings... All that, only to end up once again in the hands of neurosurgeons and oncologists, on the operating table with a big lump in my brain?

Dear reader, I feel your faith in raspberries and broccoli fading. And perhaps the same is true of your faith in physical exercise, yoga, meditation, stress management... I hear you murmuring, 'After all, if David himself, the living incarnation of this lifestyle, the one who thinks anticancer, eats anticancer, moves anticancer, breathes anticancer, *lives* anticancer – if even he succumbs to the disease, then what is left of *Anticancer*?'

Naturally, Régis wasn't the only one to ask me this question, and of course I'd already given it a lot of thought. As a matter of fact, my relapse spurred me on to ask myself a number of related questions. These are the most serious, and perhaps the most important questions of my life.

The first question I asked myself was: Are the methods that I defend in *Anticancer* still valid, or must I recognize that they don't protect against a relapse? My answer is that *Anticancer* is as valid as ever. I'll explain why later on.

But that answer immediately begs another question: Since the anticancer methods are indeed effective, why didn't they protect me? Or rather, if we agree that they have protected me since my previous relapse, why did they cease to do so, and why now? This question has forced me to do some soul-searching; to 'examine my conscience', as Catholics would say; to practise some self-criticism, as the Chinese would put it. I am forced to admit that recently I have not been the ideal embodiment of the anticancer lifestyle.

And this brings me to the third and most serious and probing question: When death comes, how will I face it? Everything I've learned in the past twenty years, all that training for the final showdown: will it stand up to the shock of reality?

I'm writing this book to address these three questions. The book is also an opportunity to say goodbye to all those who appreciated my previous books, *Healing Without Freud or Prozac* and *Anticancer*; to all those who came to listen to me speak at conferences and round-table discussions; to all those readers or listeners with whom I have so often sensed an immediate connection. I firmly hope that this goodbye will not be the last. We can say goodbye many times.

That's what I say to friends who come to see me, some times from very far away, after they learn of my relapse. When they ask, 'Will I see you again in three months?', I tell them frankly, 'I don't know.' It's sad, this ritual of bidding farewell, but it would be even worse if it were not sad. If we're lucky enough to meet again in three months' time, I'll do it again with the same pleasure and the same sadness. In the meantime, I prefer not to miss the opportunity to say goodbye to those whom I hold dear.

11

what's left of *anticancer?*

To the primary question begged by my current medical situation – 'Does my relapse undermine the credibility of the anticancer method?' – my answer is an emphatic 'No'.

I am not a scientific experiment in and of myself; I am just one clinical case among many. Scientific experiments involve data from thousands, sometimes tens of thousands of clinical cases. The recommendations, the research, the conclusions and the evidence that I present in *Anticancer* are not based on my personal experience, but on the scientific literature.

Moreover, all forms of treatment, whether they're traditional or experimental, have success and failure rates. There is no 'miracle cure' against cancer, no one hundred per cent success rate, even in conventional medicine, which is extremely effective. There is no infallible method, no surgery or chemotherapy that works every time. So it's not surprising that there is no nutritional programme, no exercise regime, no stress-management technique that has the capacity to eliminate the possibility of a relapse.

However, keeping this in mind, there are ways to maximize our natural defences by taking care of our bodies both physically and mentally. You can play all your cards right, but it still doesn't guarantee that you'll win the game.

There's no doubt that these methods, which are accessible to everyone, reinforce the potential of our natural self-defence systems. Numerous research studies have delivered conclusive proof, and fortunately there are physicians and hospitals that recognize it. When the doctors in Cologne decided I should undergo an emergency operation, not for a second did they say, 'Aha, guess your broccoli doesn't work!' On the contrary, they assured me, 'If you follow all the guidelines that you laid out in your book, you have every chance of beating this.'

I was very grateful for their attitude. Patients who mobilize their energies to reinforce their natural defences need others to recognize their efforts as worthwhile. Instead, all too often they hear: 'Do whatever you want to in terms of complementary treatment. It won't do any harm, but it may not do much good either.'

That statement is false, scientifically false. It stands for everything I've fought against. There are so many things we can legitimately do in addition to conventional medical treatment. Objectively, these 'things', which I call anticancer methods, do a great deal of good: they contribute, objectively, to improving the patient's condition; they make treatments more effective, diminish side effects, and lead to longer periods of remission and a lower risk of relapse.

For example, it has been clearly shown that physical activity helps the body tolerate chemotherapy. As a result, physicians don't need to reduce the dosages, and this directly contributes to making the chemo treatment more effective. The same applies to radiation therapy, and to recovery post-surgery. One proven effect of stress-management techniques is to reduce nausea. Anticancer methods are in reality frontline instruments for healthy living. It is unacceptable not to share that information with patients.

In my case, I am convinced that these approaches have considerably improved my life, in terms of both its span and its quality. I was first diagnosed with a brain tumour nineteen years ago. The fact that I have lived all these years with such an aggressive form of cancer – 99 per cent of people with this cancer do not live longer than six years – is enough to support the idea that it was within my power to contribute positively to my health.

At the end of *Anticancer*, I confessed that I had no idea how much time I had left to live. But whatever happened, I wrote, I was glad that I had chosen to cultivate every aspect of my health, for it had already allowed me to live a far happier life. Today, I repeat that statement. We need to nourish our health, our psychological balance, our relationships with others and the planet around us. Together, all these efforts contribute to protecting us – individually and collectively – from cancer, even if there will never be a one hundred per cent guarantee.

12

inner calm

How many times did I hear my friends say, 'Look after yourself'? They knew I was crisscrossing the globe, racing from conference to interview, and from one project to another. They worried about me doing too much. And I reassured them, saying, 'You're right, I'm going to slow down.' But I never did.

I've often said that I practised everything I recommended in *Anticancer*. For the most part, it was true. But I failed in one respect: by subjecting myself to an exhausting and ultimately excessive workload, I failed to look after myself. This overload dates back, in fact, to the publication of my previous book, *Healing Without Freud or Prozac*. I was so pleased with how well it was received that I threw myself into the promotion and defence of the ideas in the book. I got into the habit of travelling, not only in France and Europe but also in Asia, in the United States and in Canada. I subjected myself to innumerable bouts of jetlag, despite the knowledge that jetlag has a detrimental impact on the immune system because it produces stress hormones such as cortisol and upsets the body's natural cycles.

This upheaval of my biological rhythms peaked the year before my relapse. *Anticancer* was doing very well in the United States. I cared so much about promoting my ideas that I simply forgot to look after myself. In 2009 and 2010 I travelled, on average, once a month across the Atlantic, in addition to one or two trips per week in France or elsewhere in Europe. It was far too much. By the end of the year, I was utterly drained. And then the tumour reappeared.

With hindsight, I think I was driven by a very human urge to forget my condition, to feel 'normal' and to live 'like everyone else'. Above all, I think I let myself succumb to the vanity of feeling I was invincible. We must never lose our humility in the face of illness. Nobody possesses an invincible weapon against it, and the best techniques of modern medicine are fallible. Above all, we make a serious mistake if we overlook the extent to which biology is the determining factor.

Instead of remaining humble, I made the mistake of believing I had found the magic formula that would allow me to stay healthy and give myself over completely to the projects that I cared about. I told myself I was protected simply because I was still taking a certain number of precautions. I was careful about my diet, I rode my bike every day, I meditated and did some yoga. I believed that this gave me licence to ignore the fundamental needs of my body – such as sleep, rest and a regular routine.

In retrospect, my mistake is glaringly obvious. Although I may not be a one-man scientific experiment, there are some lessons to be learned here. We must not exhaust and overexert ourselves. One of the best defences against cancer is finding a place of inner calm. I realize that for people in physically demanding professions, who work at night or in shifts, this advice is hard to put into practice, just as it is for parents with young children or teenagers, or people who have to travel a great deal.

Personally, I never managed to find that calm, and today I regret it. I didn't manage to remain close to nature and to its, and my, natural rhythm. I am absolutely convinced that spending time in a forest, on a mountain or by a river-bank brings us something that is wonderfully revitalizing. Perhaps this is because it helps us to align ourselves with the rhythm of the seasons, to find balance and healing within ourselves. I don't know of any scientific studies that back up this intuition. But the idea that finding harmony with nature is good for our health is supported by a whole series of established truths.

13

priorities

I know a Canadian woman, Molly, who is roughly my age and who, like me, lives with a stage-four glioblastoma. In her case she's been living with it for about a decade, which is a truly remarkable feat. When she was first diagnosed, Molly underwent conventional treatment, and she hasn't had a relapse since. She may owe this exceptional remission to the fact that she has chosen to live in almost complete isolation north of Toronto. Every day Molly takes long walks on the banks of a lake. When you ask her, 'What is it that helps you most to keep the disease at bay?', she always responds: 'It's the quiet. The quietness protects me.'

I, on the other hand, had taken the completely opposite approach. I was convinced I did not need calm, that it was more important that I contribute to the collective wellbeing – that I help change patterns of behaviour and attitudes, with a view to creating a more balanced human ecology. I was only too happy – and I still am – to be able to participate in these advancements, and I couldn't for a second imagine giving up my life's work. But it is precisely because I found it so rewarding that I overlooked my limits. My work had become so pivotal that everything else fell by the wayside. For example, I hadn't taken a proper holiday in several years, and I almost never took time out to rest and relax. Was I wrong? It is difficult for me to judge these choices now. But if I have the chance to do it all again, I'm determined that I will no longer neglect these needs.

The notion of 'positive stress' played a role in my failure to reduce sources of tension in my life. While writing my books, I had discovered that there is a particularly fascinating variety of stress that is beneficial to the mind as well as the body. It pushes us to surpass ourselves; thanks to this stress we discover untapped resources within us and we expand our own horizons. Studies have shown that brief periods of positive stress can even reinforce our immune system.

This 'beneficial' stress is the opposite of the better-known 'negative' stress, which generates feelings of helplessness and immobility, and creates tension in the body. Experiments prove that situations of prolonged stress are highly damaging in animals, and accelerate relapses of cancer. Studies on humans show the same. We know that the feeling of helplessness weakens the immune system and causes inflammation, which encourages the growth of tumours as well as a host of other problems including heart conditions, hypertension, diabetes and arthritis.

But although 'positive' stress is undoubtedly one of the great motors driving a powerful life-force, I have come to believe that it can also act like a drug on the psyche. You can become addicted to positive stress, prompting cycles of craving and withdrawal. In particular, you can lose perspective. Perhaps that is what happened to me: I was so fulfilled and absorbed by my work that I neglected my body's needs.

This underscores how important each element of the anticancer method is in relation to the whole. Are some aspects more important than others? Are some indispensable? In *Anticancer*, I listed a large number of factors, based on scientific studies, but I never ranked them in order of importance. I wanted to allow each reader to choose, conscious that if I gave too many or overly prescriptive recommendations, I ran the risk of discouraging people rather than motivating them.

With regard to the public perception of *Anticancer*, the nutritional guidelines – such as eating raspberries, or drinking green tea – tended to overshadow other recommendations. And I myself insisted quite considerably on the nutritional aspect. It seemed to me that if people began a programme of healthy eating, it would in itself constitute enormous progress. It was also the most obvious part of the message and the simplest to apply: it's easier to eat fish and berries than it is to change your work habits or your relationship with your spouse.

*

Of course, *Anticancer* deals with other dimensions that are at least as important as nutrition, if not more so. I often wanted to clarify the question of the emphasis we should give to the various recommendations and precautions. But it's a complex subject and there is a lack of scientific data. Ultimately, each of us has to trust our instincts.

In light of my own ordeal, I'm tempted to emphasize the absolute necessity of finding and maintaining inner peace, notably through meditation, cardiac coherence exercises and a balanced lifestyle that minimizes sources of stress. Next, I would put physical exercise, whose importance cannot be overstated. And on a par with physical activity, I would put nutrition: I am glad to see that the importance of diet is now widely recognized, even by some oncologists who initially contested this idea when *Anticancer* was first published.

14

making the crossing

The third issue I'm wrestling with today is that of death itself. For twenty years I've lived with the Sword of Damocles over me, and I've been forced to think about death often. Of course, being involved in so many rewarding activities has allowed me to deflect these existential questions to some extent. But I've never really stopped asking myself, 'When *it* comes back, will I tremble with fear as I did the first time? Or will the new priorities in my life, all the essential lessons that I've learned, help me face it with composure?'

Today, when I am closer than ever to the final moment, I realize I'm reacting more or less exactly like most of the patients that I cared for as a psychiatrist: patients with cancer or other terminal illnesses who had to face the prospect of death. Like many of them, I'm afraid of suffering but I'm not afraid of dying. What I fear is dying in pain and this fear seems to me to be common to all human beings, and even to animals.

The other night I was in bed, lying on my left side –
the side that is currently disabled by the progression of
the cancer. I wanted to turn over and couldn't. I could
feel a kind of dullness numbing my body. And suddenly I
was afraid that this dullness might progress – that it might
attack my chest muscles and end up stifling my breathing.
I said to myself, 'If I can't breathe, I'll die. I'll die here,
now, tonight, like this, with nobody here, with no one
knowing what's happening.' I was terrified.

But then, quite rapidly, I realized that the numbness
wasn't actually uncomfortable at all. Compared with the
violent pain that I had suffered in previous days, it was a
gentle feeling: enveloping and gradual, similar to the sensation of being outside when it's very cold. If I was going
to die this way – rather than, say, after a year of unspeak-
able suffering – perhaps that wasn't such a bad thing. This
thought was so soothing that I fell back to sleep. When I
woke up the next morning, I was, of course, still breathing. And, most importantly, I had learned I could live
through such moments and not be at the mercy of fear.

I have often been with patients when their hope of
recovery, or of an improvement in their symptoms, gives
way to a different reality: that of imminent death. I have
been privileged to observe the way they develop another
kind of hope: the hope of dying 'well'. It's a very important challenge, and an absolutely legitimate goal. After all,
every life's journey ends in death. And I like to think, as

do many philosophers, that life is a long preparation for that supreme moment. When you stop fighting illness, you still have one challenge left: that of dying well – saying goodbye to the people to whom you need to say goodbye, forgiving those you need to forgive and asking forgiveness of those who need to forgive you. Leaving messages. Getting your affairs in order. Departing with a feeling of peace and connection.

In fact, it's a great privilege to be able to prepare your departure. With their reports of accidents and catastrophes, the evening news bulletins remind us daily that violent death can occur at any moment, abruptly wiping out its victims and depriving families of the precious chance to say goodbye.

In preparing for this crucial moment, we can call on the help of good 'allies': caregivers, legal experts and, of course, family and friends. I feel this challenge to be a crucial one, and the prospect of meeting it successfully remains a source of hope for me. What will happen afterwards, on 'the other side'? I don't know.

15

in the valley of the shadow of death

How can you not feel paralysed by fear when your prognosis is dire, the warning lights are flashing red and you are assailed by dozens of unpleasant physical symptoms all at once? This question has preoccupied me on a daily basis for the past year. I remember the day last summer when I went for lunch in Cologne with a cousin who had come to visit me. I hadn't yet recovered from my eye problems, so I asked her to read aloud for me a scientific article about the vaccine protocol I was about to embark on. The authors explained that more research was needed, since – and this was a shock to me – 'for stage-four glioblastoma, in cases of relapse the survival rate at eighteen months is zero'. A zero chance of survival beyond eighteen months! 'Those are not great odds...' It was the first time I had ever dealt with such a drastic prognosis. It was tough to swallow at lunch.

A little later my brother Franklin went to pick up the tumour that had been extracted from my brain, in order to transport it to Leuven where the vaccine was to be developed. A physician stopped short on seeing the size of my tumour. 'Is that your brother's?' he asked. 'Listen, there's no point running around the world trying out experimental treatments and research protocols. Use the time you have left to say goodbye to each other.'

Another red flag: when it was time to leave the convalescent home, my wife, who was very worried about the statistics, asked the doctors, 'What should I expect?' The registrar answered in a friendly voice, 'The way things are right now, I'd advise you to take each day as a gift, and try not to think about anything else.'

There were also the visits of two kind ministers, one in the hospital, the other at the convalescent home. They came to the rooms with their portable altar folded in a black pouch. They were both Protestant, but they each managed to bring me a Communion wafer 'borrowed' from a Catholic priest. And they both proposed to read to me the celebrated Psalm 23, attributed to David, 'The Lord Is My Shepherd':

> *The Lord is my shepherd; I shall not want*
> *He maketh me to lie down in green pastures:*
> *He leadeth me beside the still waters.*
> *He restoreth my soul:*
> *He leadeth me in the paths of righteousness for his*
>   *name's sake.*

Yea, though I walk through the valley of the shadow
*   of death, I will fear no evil:*
For thou art with me;
Thy rod and thy staff, they comfort me.
Thou preparest a table before me in the presence of
*   mine enemies,*
Thou anointest my head with oil; my cup runneth
*   over.*
Surely goodness and mercy shall follow me all the
*   days of my life*
And I will dwell in the house of the Lord, for ever.

If a priest comes to see you with this, the 'pearl of psalms', which also happens to be the psalm of death, it's not a good sign. It means he's been briefed, and the medical team is not optimistic. Still, I was delighted to receive the visit of the chaplains, and that psalm became my shield against fear.

When you find yourself at such an advanced stage of illness, and when the prognosis is so bleak, there are childish, irrational – primitive, perhaps – fears that surge up from the depths of your psyche. You find yourself surrounded by strange shadows, ominous signs, sinister noises. For a few months now, I've been noticing that this fear takes on surprising forms. As I go to sleep, I am haunted by the fear that I will be attacked by vampires and werewolves. I must have been eight years old the last time these malevolent creatures made me tremble in terror. But now they're back to inhabit my nights.

I can easily guess what's hiding behind these folkloric remnants: the fear of what's in store for me, the thing that's pursuing me and that wants to cut my life short. Despite being able to coldly analyse my emotions, and though I feel no conscious fear at the possibility of death, when night falls I make sure that I have a can of Mace close to my working hand, in case one of those predators comes too close to my bedside... And when scary shapes streak across the walls of my room, I repeat to myself variations of the verses of Psalm 23: 'You are walking through the valley of the shadow of death. And what you're seeing are the shadows of death. But you need fear no evil, for the Lord is your shepherd. His hand is in yours, and he will always be there with you.' I'm not entirely sure I believe in that providential, divine shepherd, but this psalm has a powerfully calming effect on my nocturnal torments.

Ever since cancer entered my life, another thought has always been immensely helpful and continues to soothe my soul. It's the knowledge that I'm not the only one who will die. It's not as though I was being unfairly punished, thrown into a dungeon on bread and water rations. No. Everyone will go through it one day.

It's sad that my time will come sooner, but it's not a monstrous injustice. I've been blessed in my life: I've had some extraordinary encounters, I have known what it is to love, I have had children, I have had exceptional brothers and friends, I have left my mark. I've lived through many deeply enriching experiences, and cancer has been one of them. I haven't let my life slip through my fingers. And if it all ends at the age of fifty, or fifty-one, or fifty-two, that's not so tragic. Living to the age of eighty without achieving any of my hopes and dreams – now *that* would have broken my heart.

When I bring this up with my oncologist, he looks concerned and suggests I see a psychiatrist. As if I might be surrendering to fatalism and despair. However, this is not the case. I'm still fighting for my health. I'm simply convinced that being at peace with yourself, and accepting your mortality, means you can direct all your energy towards the healing process.

16

no regrets

Recently, Franklin and Edouard came to me with a question I found particularly difficult. 'If, four years ago, someone had told you that if you kept on living at the same pace you would be heading straight for a relapse, this time with a much more aggressive tumour, would you have lived any differently?'

I answered as sincerely as I could. 'No. Strange as it may seem, no. I prefer the path I took, even if it's brought me to the edge of a cliff.'

My answer stunned them. 'You admit that you seriously neglected the basic needs of your body, you say that you're ready to change everything, and yet you still would have chosen the same crazy path?'

It's contradictory, I admit, and maybe it does seem mad. My brothers don't understand these choices, and they chastise me for not having taken better care of my health. They're right, of course. But my position isn't as incoherent as it might appear. I am, indeed, aware that I'm up against it, and I'm determined to change a lot of things about my life. I've already begun. But when I look back, how can I overlook how much I've loved my work, and what unforgettable satisfaction it has brought me? How could I reject that driving force, even though it might have played a part in causing this relapse?

I've tried to explain my choices by referring to my favourite sports. They are activities that you might characterize as 'extreme': surfing, paragliding, canyoneering, skiing, that kind of thing. What I like about these sports isn't only that they put you in touch with nature, but more specifically that they are subject to the elements – the wind, the waves, the currents – and it is to these that you must submit. You can't claim to control anything: you throw yourself into the water or into the wind, and then you try to navigate and adapt to what nature throws at you. This high degree of uncertainty, this 'by the grace of God' aspect, suits my character, and I embrace the unpredictability and the risks. With these sports there is a wager of acceptance, a need to adapt to the world as it is, a humility even, which in some respects reminds me of the teachings of Eastern philosophy.

I must confess that I sometimes find myself considering my relapse as another stimulating, almost invigorating challenge. It's as if a very big wave had crashed into my routine and plunged me into a raging sea. All of a sudden I'm forced to ask myself a number of essential questions, to make radical changes, to explore uncharted territory, while fighting to keep my head above water. Whatever the outcome, it will have been a thrilling adventure.

This is not to imply that I feel no fear. I'm scared as hell. But at the same time I feel a kind of excitement. Perhaps I'm addicted to adrenalin and the tsunami of hormones it sets off in my body. Having been forced for so long to face an illness that is by definition terminal, I've been fighting most of my life, and I've known the dangerous high of those who think they've conquered fate. In the end, biology always has the last word, and it's rather arrogant to forget it. But these intense struggles have given me a perhaps excessive taste for extreme and difficult challenges.

On a more intellectual level, this tendency was fuelled by the sometimes epic battles that I fought to defend the positions I took in *Healing Without Freud or Prozac* and *Anticancer*. These confrontations charged my life with meaning, as if I were permanently wired up to an electrical outlet. I was driven by such an intense sense of purpose that it was impossible for me to let go.

And now I am obliged to address these uncomfortable questions. Did I push myself too far? Did I set the right priorities for myself? Did I lead a worthwhile life, and does it deserve to be continued? If so, under what conditions? If I were to change it, where would I begin? I hope I have time to find the answers.

17

a lesson in courage

My father, Jean-Jacques, had his own personal methods for teaching us how to be brave. I remember one trip to Florida. Every evening, at the time of day when the sea is calmest, he took me out on a boat to teach me how to water-ski. I knew there were sharks in the area. This was nerve-racking enough by day; at night, it was downright terrifying. But sharks or no sharks, I had to jump into the water unless I wanted my father to throw me in. He wasn't scared of sharks. I just had to follow his example.

My father explained that sharks would far rather eat fish than children, and accidents rarely occur. He thought it was worth taking a few risks for the sake of water-skiing. Needless to say, I was highly motivated to get up out of the water at lightning speed, concentrate on keeping my balance and learn as quickly as possible how not to fall. There's nothing more terrifying than skiing at dusk on dark waters, where you think you can make out the shadow of a shark. Nothing, not even a serious relapse of your cancer.

I was twelve or thirteen the first time my father took me heli-skiing in the Pyrenees. A helicopter flew us high into the mountains and dropped us off at the top of a glacier. We had to ski down it, avoiding the numerous crevasses and the debris beneath the snow. That was the whole appeal of heli-skiing. At one point, one of my skis hit a large rock. My ski came off, and I tumbled perhaps fifty yards. I was scared. But the next time it happened I was less frightened. When you've been through danger and survived it, you're not as petrified by it. You can learn to be brave.

This is exactly what my father – who was known for his daring – had wanted. But my father wasn't only a courageous athlete (though he did enjoy extreme skiing in avalanche zones). Around 1940, when he was at school in the French alpine city of Grenoble, he climbed the façade of the school and unhooked the swastika flag that hung above the entrance. He was fifteen years old, and wore a pair of British army shorts. Every time I have had to face adversity, the idea that I have his blood in my veins, and that I was shaped by his daredevil spirit, has been a great help to me. I'm still horribly frightened, of course; but I know how to avoid becoming paralysed by fear. The kind of courage my father taught me is about holding your ground when you're shaking like a leaf; it's not about pretending that you're not afraid.

Having been trained in this school of valour (that verged on recklessness), it was only normal that in my childhood I should encounter a few setbacks. At the age of twelve, for example, during a skiing trip, a friend and I decided to do some improvised slaloming between enormous telegraph poles. I smashed my femur on a steel pole after slipping on a patch of ice. Three months of enforced immobility certainly tried my patience, but it didn't make me any less reckless afterwards.

At fifteen I did something just as stupid, but this time I paid a higher price. Disappointed at having lost a swimming race, I decided to console myself by going riding. But the only horse available had not been broken in, and was standing in a field with only a rope around its neck. Of uncertain pedigree, this creature had developed the habit of getting rid of any riders by racing hell-for-leather towards an obstacle and then stopping dead. I knew all this, but the urge was too strong for me to resist.

I had scarcely managed to clamber onto his back when he took off, racing headlong towards an apple tree. I thought to myself, 'I know what you've got in mind; you're not going to be done with me that easily,' and clung onto his neck. But you can't control an untamed horse when you've got no saddle, no stirrups and no reins. When he reached the tree I was ejected like a cannon ball. I somersaulted through the air and came crashing down right against the tree trunk. I could have been killed. Fortunately my leg took most of the impact. I found myself lying under the tree, with my left foot grotesquely splayed in front of

my nose. I was in blinding pain. It was a severe open frac-
ture. I yelled, but I was too far from the path for anyone
to hear me. After an hour that felt more like an eternity, a
friend of mine found me and alerted my parents.

My father was unhappy to see me suffering, of course.
But he didn't scold me. He didn't say, 'Can't you be a
bit more careful?' The way he saw it, this kind of unfor-
tunate experience was just one of the unavoidable risks of
living. My father was convinced that taking a few knocks
was character-building. Ever since his training as a fighter
pilot, he had retained a military attitude and an endless
fascination for structure, hierarchy, missions and objectives.
Ideologically, however, he was anti-military, and above all
anti-colonialist. These ideals led him to enlist in another
war, this time as the co-founder and editor-in-chief of the
weekly magazine *L'Express*, taking the lead in a heated
campaign against France's role in the war in Algeria (where
he had courageously fought, albeit against his will), and
against the use of torture. He didn't merely denounce an
unjust war: he firmly lobbied for the elimination of conscrip-
tion, which 'wasted too much time for too many people'.

I was shaped, the hard way, by this passionate man
bursting with contradictions, whose life, over the years,
had become a source of inspiration and a moral compass
for me. Seeing my father speak in public and defend his
ideas before rowdy audiences helped me immensely when
I in turn faced my own critics. I learned early on that these

battles are not part of the game – these are not playful subjects – but part of the effort, part of what it takes to achieve the goals you set for yourself.

Even the stories about my father that I know only from hearsay made a lasting impression on me. I remember a fairly serious accident that happened one day when I was paragliding. The wind dropped abruptly, and I saw a little copse of trees coming up towards me fast. I thought I'd have just enough room to glide over it, before suddenly realizing that no – I was no longer high enough. As I watched a tree approach at such alarming speed that I was clearly destined to hit it, images of my father as a young fighter pilot crashing into a forest flashed through my mind. When he was barely twenty years old, he had been recruited into the Free French forces to be trained by the US Air Force in Alabama, and one day he had an accident. As his P-47 collided with the trees, branches broke off in quick succession against the wings, finally bringing his aircraft to a halt. It required some acrobatics for my father to pull himself from the wreckage. But he survived, just as I survived that paragliding accident.

Now that I, too, am a father, I admit that it worries me when my son Sacha takes risks. But I would also be worried if he didn't take any. I need to be reassured that he is courageous, that something of my father's daring has been passed on to him through me. He doesn't need to take on the Nazis of today. Seeing him ride horses or surf is enough to bring me joy and pride; in that regard, my wishes have been entirely fulfilled. I remember the first time I took him paragliding, at the age of eight. With his instructor behind him, he had to run to the edge of a precipice and jump off into the void. I was standing below him, at a good angle to take photos, and at the moment he took off I could clearly see the incredible expression of elation that lit up his face. I was very proud that day. Sacha had had the guts to dive in without hesitating or asking too many questions. In fact, he would have been furious if I had prevented him from doing it. At eight years old, that's pretty good.

I hope that I can be an example for my two other children, Charlie and Anna, as my father was for me. I hope they can retain an image of me that will help shape them when I'm no longer present, just as I was shaped by the image of my father. I have been able to take care of Charlie, who was born two years before my relapse, but Anna came into the world in the middle of the storm; I've never been able to look after her. I hope, however, that I can leave them both a little of that determination that has got me through my toughest moments. And, most importantly, the conviction that if they give themselves wholeheartedly to their chosen goals, they can hope to go far.

18

comrades in arms

I often think of my friend Bernard Giraudeau, who died of cancer last summer, just as I was beginning my own battle against this relapse. Bernard was both a companion in my struggle and a role model. I admired the way he'd been able to abandon the insatiable habits of his notoriously excessive lifestyle, and to concentrate, ultimately, on a new way of life, mercilessly casting aside everything that he judged to be unimportant or futile. A true hedonist, Bernard loved to laugh and he had developed a science of pleasure; I have always tended to take things a little too seriously, but some of Bernard's *joie de vivre* rubbed off on me.

Bernard had decided that it was crucial to relax, to take holidays, to relish the present moment, to have a 'good' life. I especially remember the summer of 2006, on the Ile de Ré, an island off the western coast of France where we saw each other often. I was staying at my dear friend Madeleine Chapsal's house in the village of Les Portes en Ré, where Bernard also had a home. We would sometimes meditate together in the early morning and then go swimming. I'm certain that in order to savour life to the very end, as Bernard did, you first need to make peace with yourself, and with death.

The example of the French-Canadian psychoanalyst Guy Corneau has also been an enormous inspiration. Two years ago Guy was diagnosed with a very serious cancer: a lymphoma in the stomach, spleen and lungs. But thanks to a strict programme that combined conventional treatment with complementary methods such as meditation, visualization and energy therapy, he is now in remission.

Guy laughed as he told me the story of how, when his oncologist had told him that he had a stage-four lymphoma, he hadn't thought to ask how many stages there were. It was only afterwards, when he knew he would survive, that he asked, 'So, how many stages are there?' And the doctor said, 'Four. You were at death's door.'

Guy believes that your mental state is crucial. He reacted to his diagnosis by radically changing his lifestyle: he created a healthy environment, eliminated sources of stress and chose to live close to nature. To be able to focus on his treatments, he stopped working, devoting his time fully to meditation and visualization. Of course, not everyone is in a position to do this. Not only was Guy able to make that choice, but he did so by applying his new rules for life with total determination. Today all traces of his tumour have disappeared and he has started working again part-time, but he remains intent on not forgetting the lessons he learned from cancer.

Like Bernard, like Guy, I am certain that when you're in the advanced stages of cancer, one of your most urgent tasks is to find and preserve a degree of calm without which your mental and physical state will crumble. One of the things that has helped me the most in this respect is meditation. I know that for most people this word conjures up incense, trippy music and Tibetan monks sitting in the lotus position on a mountain-top. Though it's true that many Tibetan monks in remote monasteries do indeed practise advanced spiritual exercises, meditation is something we can all do. We mere mortals can also, at our own pace and level, learn to practise this discipline with a more modest goal: improving our health.

19

prescription: laughter and meditation

The positive effects of meditation have been so clearly demonstrated that hundreds of hospitals in the United States as well as increasing numbers in Europe now teach their patients a method developed by a famous American molecular biologist, Jon Kabat-Zinn. His method draws on yoga, Zen and practices related to Tibetan Buddhism. I've been practising this method, which is called 'mindfulness', for many years, with a few breaks that always make it slightly hard work to start up again. But overall, I've found ways to set aside fifteen or twenty minutes twice a day for this vital exercise.

I remember when Charlie was born, and I used to get up in the morning to change his nappy and give him a bottle: I loved having his company afterwards for my meditation session. Sitting in his baby walker, he would watch me practise yoga, followed by twenty minutes of meditation. It can't be much fun for a baby to watch his father meditate.

But Charlie's patience was angelic. I suppose he was waiting for the far more amusing moment when I would switch to abdominal crunches. Every time I raised my torso up towards him, he would burst into happy giggles.

Mindfulness is a common concept in Buddhism, but Kabat-Zinn has purged it of any religious reference. As he teaches it, mindfulness means centring on yourself and your breathing. It's not narcissism. The process is not about giving yourself an ego-boost. The objective is to attain the highest level of physical self-awareness by focusing on the act of breathing. In so doing, we gradually rid ourselves of thoughts until we have as few as possible. The result is an extremely restful state where we are in fact momentarily released from the tyranny of our ego. This state could be described as the physical sensation of being yourself, at peace.

I usually practise mindfulness twice a day, morning and evening, sitting comfortably on a meditation cushion filled with rice or grains of spelt, my spine as straight as possible to make it easier to concentrate on the physical sensations. At the moment my legs are very weak and I find it difficult to cross them. When I'm too tired, I meditate lying down. But that position is less conducive to concentration. When I focus on my breathing, on the quality of my inhalations and exhalations, my thoughts slowly subside and I am overcome with a feeling of infinite calm. The purpose of meditation is not to reach a 'pleasant' state of being. Everyone who meditates will say that, and they're right. But it seems to me that the fact that it *is* pleasant really helps motivate us to do it and encourages us to do it regularly.

I realize that meditation remains very abstract if you haven't tried it. Kabat-Zinn addresses people who argue that they don't have the time or the energy by saying, 'The more problems you have, the more you need to meditate. The more complicated your life is, the more you need to meditate – to help you manage the problems and complications.' Personally, I no longer question the time commitment, because I know that the few minutes I devote to mindfulness are paid back to me a hundred times over in terms of my mental and physical wellbeing. It's like having a dog: you take it out every morning without even thinking about it, whether it's raining or windy, whether you're up to your neck in work or have nothing else to do. Meditation is a bit like that. No matter what happens, you know you need to give yourself fresh air every day.

Recently, inspired by Guy Corneau, I've been trying to incorporate visualization exercises into my meditation. This is a more 'active' method than mindfulness: it consists of visualizing negative thoughts, such as fear or anger, in the form of black smoke that you exhale with every breath. Conversely, as you breathe in you try to inhale white, or 'positive', 'invigorating' colours: bright yellows, reds and blues. This ancient Buddhist technique was taught to me by a Tibetan doctor living in Paris. The goal of the exercise is to 'clean' the negative emotions by exhaling them, until the smoke becomes white, vibrant and joyful.

In the Tibetan tradition, this method is not considered to be 'spiritual'. Its aim is not to bring the practitioner closer to his or her Buddha nature, for example. It's an exercise of mental yoga, which is said to help fight all kinds of illnesses; a sort of generic Tibetan medicine, in the purest mind–body tradition. Its mode of action isn't to target and attack some specific pathological factor at work in a particular disease; it is to give broad assistance to the innate processes that 'build' health.

I try to practise this method every day, even though I find the visualization exercises more difficult than the familiar serenity of mindfulness. More generally, I try now to remain as connected as possible to my inner feelings: attentive to the little emotional shifts that signify the build-up of tension, or a fleeting moment of joy. It's important to have deep knowledge of your own inner landscape, so that you know at every moment whether you're in a zone of serenity or a zone of stress – and you know when the shift occurs, and why. I try to discern and detect the sources of tension, and I learn to avoid them as much as possible.

At the same time I seek to identify the emotional sources that reduce tension and I draw on them as much as I can. This requires a lot of attention, concentration and determination. For a long time I directed all my energy towards action; now I'm learning step by step to explore the secret garden of calm. I've got a long way to go, given my starting point, but I'm making headway.

20

nurturing
appreciation

Rachel Naomi Remen, an author I admire, shares in her book *Kitchen Table Wisdom* the story of a woman who has cancer and goes to chemotherapy sessions alone. On her way home, she sometimes feels so ill that she has to pull over to throw up at the side of the road. Rachel asks her, 'Why don't you have a friend come with you?' 'My friends aren't doctors or nurses,' the woman explains. 'They don't know anything about this stuff. It's not worth bothering them.' But Rachel responds that of course they can help, by easing the feelings of isolation and sadness. A child who has fallen and scraped her knee needs more than antiseptic or sticking plasters; she needs her mother to console her. A mother's kiss, like a friend's presence, doesn't heal the physical wound, but it lessens the emotional pain.

During the difficult days in Cologne when I was convalescing after my operation, many friends came to visit, some to share a meal, others to spend a few hours or a day with me. They weren't doctors, but their presence brought me great comfort. It's not so hard to talk to someone who's fighting illness. You have to listen with your heart and say, quite simply, 'I'm sorry for what you're going through. It makes me very sad. I hope you get better soon. Tell me what I can do to help.' Sometimes a small physical gesture, like putting your hand on their hand, or on their shoulder, is enough. The act of touching says very directly, 'I'm here with you. I know you're suffering. It's important for me to be here for you.'

I remember, in the days immediately following the operation, receiving a phone call from my cousin Pascaline. I was still extremely tired and I needed to sleep a great deal to regain my strength. Pascaline was calling from the other side of the world, though, so my brother decided to wake me. I spoke to her only briefly, but she told me everything I needed to hear: 'I want you to follow your treatments. I'm counting on you to get through this, because I love you and I need you in my life. It's hard for me to see you go through this ordeal, but I think you're going to make it.' She didn't speak for long, but what she said was perfect.

It's difficult to retain your sense of dignity when you become disabled and bedridden. You become dependent on others for even the most mundane things, like putting on your underpants. You lose your privacy. And here too it's important to know how to say simple things like: 'I hope it doesn't bother you too much if I do this or that?' Of course, sometimes it's necessary to move quickly; sometimes, for example, you have to hurry up with the shower because a meal is on its way. The danger for the caregiver is doing things merely mechanically; but there's nothing mechanical about the experience for the person who is naked, and who dreads above all being treated like an infant or an animal.

The patient also needs to recognize that his or her family has to adapt to the situation. Nobody is accustomed to giving a shower to an adult, or to helping him or her go to the toilet, even if that person is a husband, a brother or a mother. The family members who drop everything to come to the aid of their sick loved one need to feel that they are respected and that their help and care are not taken for granted.

When this 'family etiquette' is followed by both sides, and the patient feels well cared for and beloved, the danger of sinking into despair diminishes. Nowadays the most innovative research in psychology focuses on a state which is extremely beneficial for health, both physical and mental, and which was neglected for a long time: optimism. My recipe for preserving my optimism is to concentrate on what's going well. Every day, I take stock of and appreciate all the things, large and small, which have been agreeable, or have brought me pleasure, joy or simply amusement. I consciously cultivate my feeling of gratitude. I don't have to make a huge effort: I adore eating, I really like good food, and I'm fortunate to have excellent and completely 'anticancer' meals lovingly prepared for me by my dear Liliane, who has been caring for my family for fifty years. I also love listening to music. And I love seeing movies and re-watching classics. I love meeting new people, and then seeing them again. There are many things I enjoy every day. I'm very lucky.

21

precious moments

When you lose hope, everything stops, including the desire to continue with the very treatment that might be your only chance of survival. As far as I'm concerned, I continue to live with the hope that although my symptoms are serious, they will get better. I devote a lot of my energy to nourishing my spirit and the spark of life within me, to strengthening my muscles, alleviating my headaches, staying calm. I work on remaining connected with my loved ones and try to focus on everything that gives me pleasure in life. I cultivate these sources of hope very attentively. They give me the desire to live until tomorrow and the day after tomorrow and the day after that. I'm convinced that we need to do everything possible to help patients preserve their ability to hope. It's not a question of telling white lies: you don't have to distort the truth to give someone hope.

One source of hope, when disability becomes intolerable and your general condition is deteriorating, is the pleasure that you feel in the company of close family and friends. In my case, just seeing my wife and children will make my day, but even a pet can illuminate the drab landscape of disease. Many years ago, I had to endure a gruelling course of chemotherapy that lasted thirteen months. I found an unorthodox way to calm my terrible nausea: I would sleep beside my dog, and stroke him from time to time. It was as if my dog understood that he had a role to play in helping me recover. Every morning I went running with him. Or rather, since he took his mission to heart, it would be more accurate to say that every morning he took *me* running.

This is obviously something my cat, Titus, can't do. But he keeps me company very faithfully, and each night gives me the great gift of sleeping curled against my legs. Thank you, Titus: with you I feel less alone in the dark.

Alongside these sources of joy there are also the little pleasures of life, and the most gratifying to me have always been physical activities. The idea that I will probably have to give up all the sports that I love – cycling, surfing, paragliding – makes me extremely sad. Even walking has become difficult. Nowadays I have to content myself with more passive pleasures, like watching a good film or chatting with friends. I know I am lucky to have them. The fact that I enjoy eating is encouraging. When your appetite disappears, due to nausea and a shrunken stomach, your desire to live takes a bad hit.

Another of life's little pleasures that I hold very dear is laughter. The first time I had cancer, one of the few people who knew of my diagnosis happened to see me in the street, laughing with my brother. He shot me a glaring look that seemed to say, 'How dare he laugh when he's just learned he has brain cancer?' That look in his eyes sent chills down my spine. I thought, 'If I have to stop laughing just because I have cancer, then I'm dead already.' I understood that you should never, absolutely never, let go of the most precious faculty of all, which is the ability to laugh with all your heart. Even when you're suffering from a fatal illness, there are still plenty of reasons to laugh, and I strongly recommend that as they fly past you, you reach out and grasp every one you can.

22

lourdes

In 2001, when I left my post at the hospital in Pittsburgh to return to France, my friends and colleagues who were aware of my cancer diagnosis made me swear I would go to Lourdes. In the United States, this Catholic pilgrimage is held in high esteem, and the idea that you might find yourself in southwest France and *not* visit the cave in the Pyrenees where Bernadette Soubirous experienced her revelations is inconceivable.

Although I agreed to bring them back some water from Lourdes, I didn't immediately keep my word. In the end, it happened more or less by accident. My brother Edouard and I had gone to the Pyrenees with the intention of going paragliding together, but the wind had grown too strong and we said to each other, 'Why not make a quick trip to Lourdes?' That's how I discovered an approach to health that cleverly taps into one's inner resources.

The pilgrimage provokes powerful emotions – anxiety, trust, surprise, feelings of communion – which are reinforced by the general atmosphere of introspection, religious fervour and expectancy. All this is magnified by the intense sensory experiences that are part of the ritual itself. In short, you find in Lourdes an impressive example of mind–body synergy.

The ritual begins with a confession. You take a ticket and wait your turn in an enormous room that looks like a railway station. There are rows of confessionals, with signs indicating the language spoken by the priest in attendance. (Almost every language is available.) When it's your turn, you have a brief conversation with a priest who explains how you can make the most of your visit. Then you suffer a little, waiting in the hot sun, before you go into the building that houses the pool: it's time to prepare yourself for the key moment of the pilgrimage. You get undressed except for a simple towel. Everyone is shivering, and not just because it's suddenly so cool after the baking sun outside – a crowd of unclothed people huddling together can conjure up sinister images. The act of making oneself 'naked before the Lord' also triggers a rare and very intense emotion, one of both humility and trust. Two volunteer attendants then take you and plunge you suddenly into the freezing water while intoning prayers aloud. It's a vertiginous and unsettling moment, to say the least.

The purification ritual comes to a close at the end of the day with a very moving grand procession followed by a mass, which is, if I recall correctly, in Latin, with subtitles provided in several languages on a screen. Everyone joins in, chanting the prayers. It's impossible not to be moved by this devotion, this personal and intimate quest combining suffering and faith. While I was among this fervent congregation, I sensed an unusual energy, at once humbling and imbued with a powerful dimension of connection to others, and directed completely towards the hope of a cure.

That short trip made a lasting impression on me, and I would like to be able to return. The doctor in me can't help but see it as an excellent investment in health: it's accessible, practically free, has no side effects whatsoever, and when it works, it *really* works. There is of course no guarantee, but then again, no treatment is guaranteed to work. Above all, this ritual, honed by almost one hundred and fifty years of practice, is a prime example of how we can take advantage of our innate capacity to heal.

23

breaking the silence

During the many years I worked as a psychiatrist in the United States, I practised not in a psychiatric hospital, where people with mental illness are treated, but in a general hospital, where the patients were suffering from all kinds of physical illnesses. Hospitals are also, in our developed countries, the place where people are brought towards the end of their lives. These patients are often dealing with excruciating pain, persistent nausea, the loss of control over their bodies, and often show signs of anxiety, depression and suicidal feelings. In these cases, the psychiatrist is called in as a matter of course. Rather than waste time on abstract intellectual theories, I would immediately begin by focusing on the patients' physical discomfort. Once they were given the right medication, and if I followed up with daily visits, their psychological state improved almost naturally.

I used this approach with many of my patients in the terminal stages of their illnesses. I saw their conditions deteriorate, I saw them go from bad to worse, and yet, when the end came, they died peacefully. I would go so far as to say that they had a 'good' death and that, at the moment they passed away, they seemed somehow happy. I believe that most of them saw death as a transition, a passage from the life we know to something else that we cannot know. A transition similar to birth, but going the other way.

These examples have often encouraged and even consoled me. They demonstrate that suffering doesn't have to be a part of death, contrary to the widely held belief that death hurts, that 'passing through the narrow gate' is inherently painful. People think of the well-documented grimace on a dying person's face, which they interpret as an expression of suffering. In reality, at the moment of death, all the muscles contract and the facial muscles do briefly form this grimace. But then, as I have witnessed many times, the face soon relaxes into an expression of peace. Death is not painful in and of itself; it often comes softly, similar to falling asleep.

That said, many terminal illnesses can be extremely painful, and relieving that suffering should be a priority. Thankfully, modern medicine now has the means to ease nearly all pain. Caregivers need to make an effort to find the right treatment, but once it has been found, pain is no longer an unavoidable curse. The problem with these medications, of course, is that at high doses they can lead to mental confusion and erode a patient's sense of themselves and their surroundings. Many patients understandably fear the side effects of these substances. They need all their mental clarity to continue to experience the love and support of their family, or to be able to bid them farewell. But on the whole, these days physicians know how to administer drugs and manage pain effectively, which is reassuring.

My experience has led me to believe that in order to confront illness as best you can, you need to think about death. This question haunts anyone who suffers from a terminal disease like cancer, even if they don't talk about it. As soon as someone says, 'I have cancer, I'm undergoing such and such a treatment,' death is in the picture. It's impossible to deny it. I'm convinced that it's better to put the subject on the table and consider it from all angles, practical and symbolic, so that when the time comes, it can happen in the best possible way. At that point, it is the most fundamental subject in the patient's life, and he or she wants to get it right.

At the same time, the simple fact of discussing it may give the patient the impression – often mistaken – that his or her end is imminent, and this can lead to enormous anxiety. The family might therefore prefer to avoid the subject as long as the person's health is not too bad. But then it's often too late, as the patient is no longer in a state to be able to discuss or even think about it.

My dialogue with patients has taught me that there is no 'good' moment to address the subject. You can do it whenever you want, so long as you don't overwhelm the patient, or give them the impression that 'it's over'. It's also better to remain vague and nuanced, even if that isn't always easy. Yes, death may come, but it's not a done deal and a cure is never out of the question.

During daily visits with patients who were nearing the end of their lives, I would slowly prepare for the moment when I would be able to ask, 'Have you thought about what could happen if the treatment isn't successful?' This opened the door to a discussion about their death, which allowed me to evaluate their level of anxiety and to determine whether there were fears we could try to defuse.

For certain fragile personalities, thinking about their own death is unimaginable. It is quite literally beyond their strength, and they should not be forced to talk about it. But these cases are rare. I've found that the vast majority of patients welcome the question almost with relief. Of course death frightens them, but they don't want to burden their close friends and family with it, so they keep their worries to themselves. They are waiting for someone to give them permission to talk about it.

Once the taboo is broken, the atmosphere doesn't need to become morbid. You can immediately bounce back, watch a light comedy, tell silly jokes, share a good meal, and above all, continue to live. It's not helpful to dwell on the subject constantly; it would be like receiving the last rites every day!

24

looking to the future

The grimmest and probably most difficult task, if you are a parent, is making decisions about your children's future. You have to be able to sit down with your partner and say, 'You know, I have something difficult I want to talk to you about... I don't know how much longer I'll still be here. We're kidding ourselves if we pretend everything is going to be fine. There are certain things we can plan for the children's future now. If you're OK with it, I'd like you to know that it would help me to talk about it and to be assured that everything is in place. You're the only one who can help me do this.' It's a distressing conversation but profoundly reassuring at the same time, as I can attest. Knowing I might not be around to watch my children grow up, that I might not be able to protect them, is heartbreaking. The only thing that comforts me is the knowledge that they have a wonderful mother who will love and take care of them.

In these highly emotional moments, it is important to avoid falling into the trap of pathos, and overdoing it.

Certainly you can talk about the pain of those who are left behind. But too much pathos might lead to dark thoughts, which are not helpful and can be damaging. Focusing on the practical aspect is, on the contrary, very beneficial, because concrete action is always preferable to negative ruminations. You can discuss the funeral, where you wish to be buried, your last will and testament. Making these decisions is far less stressful than you might imagine.

I was surprised to discover how rewarding it can be to write a last will and testament. It gives you a sense of total control, as well as a feeling of generosity, of giving, of leaving a legacy. I remember a hilarious conversation that I had recently with Edouard, when we drew up the playlist of music to be played – though I'm not in any hurry to listen to it! – while I die.

I must confess that I've fallen into the habit of thinking about my burial, but not in any macabre way. If I dared, I would almost write the script of my funeral. The benevolence of those in attendance, the kindness of their words, the general atmosphere of goodwill. No more aggressive polemics, no more gratuitous attacks. It would be the high point of my life, a kind of apotheosis. What a pity that I'll be the only one who can't attend! I haven't given in to the temptation to dictate my instructions quite yet, as I suppose I'm not the best person to handle those details.

My long experience in accompanying the dying has probably toughened me up to the terror of death, but I haven't forgotten that you can lose all your composure when that final hour comes. While I've seen many people slip away peacefully, I have also at times watched others – who were just as courageous – die an anguished death. There's no reason this couldn't happen to me; it would be arrogant to pretend otherwise. And I ask my family not to hold it against me, should they see me trembling when I reach death's door.

25

emily's breath

Emily, who died at the age of twenty-four, has been a kind of guardian angel for many years, a benevolent presence watching over my life. She was a wonderful young woman whom I had the privilege of treating when I was a psychiatrist in Pittsburgh many years ago. She suffered from a very rare form of cancer – a tumour of the adrenal glands that had entered the vena cava and invaded her heart. She was pretty, radiant, sweet, very smart and extremely generous, and was studying at Harvard when she learned she was ill. Her major was Education, and although she was the heiress to one of the greatest fortunes in Pittsburgh, she wanted to work in schools in underprivileged neighbourhoods after graduation. She was also a terrific athlete and a rowing champion.

During the last months of Emily's life I was fortunate to meet with her often. I helped her as best I could to heal residual psychic scars caused by traumas in her childhood.

We worked with hypnosis and EMDR* therapy. Despite the fear of dying and her physical pain, she maintained a profound serenity and an exceptional capacity to look out for others right to the end. It was surprising to see – almost staggering: she was dazzling, she glowed like a saint. I wasn't the only one to feel respect and infinite gratitude towards her. All those who knew Emily have the impression that in some mysterious way she has kept contact with the people who helped her at the end of her life, and that wherever she is now, she's trying in turn to help them through their own trials.

Following a risky operation that almost cost her her life, Emily remained in an intensive care unit for a long time, until her condition stabilized. Later she shared with me her extraordinary experience of when she was hovering between life and death. She had very clear memories of it. She was in a tunnel, and at the end of this tunnel was a soothing white light that drew her towards it. But it wasn't her time, and with regret she had to turn back and return to her poor, damaged body.

Four or five of my patients have told me of similar experiences. They did so spontaneously, without my asking them. Initially I knew nothing of such phenomena – at the time they were completely absent from the curriculum of

* Eye-movement desensitization and reprocessing, discussed further in my first book, *Healing Without Freud or Prozac*.

medical studies. We know more about them today; it's esti-
mated that between 8 and 15 per cent of the population,
depending on the country, have experienced this kind of
extreme state known as near-death experience (NDE). The
number is increasing, if only because of the improvement
in resuscitation techniques following cardiac arrest, which
means more and more lives can be saved. The term 'near-
death' is in fact not terribly accurate, for most of these
patients have actually experienced clinical death before
'returning to life'. They are quite literally resuscitated.

Since the pioneering work in the 1970s by the
Swiss psychiatrist Elisabeth Kübler-Ross and the American doctor Raymond Moody, research into this subject has
multiplied. Several hypotheses – ranging from hallucin-
ation to the existence of a consciousness that can survive
death – have been put forward to explain NDE. But all
the studies agree on one point: regardless of ethnic or religious origin, regardless of the historical era (the Myth of
Er in Plato may be the most ancient account of this), and
no matter what interpretation is given to the experience
by the individual in question, certain factors are almost
always present: the passage towards light, the light of love;
the feeling of peace and celestial joy; deceased relatives and
friends waiting at the end of the tunnel; the desire to stay
with them; and the reluctance to return.

My patients too had gone through episodes of clinical death, but been yanked back to life by the unstinting

efforts of their medical teams. Generally, their physical condition had suffered: it's not actually terribly good for you to die, even if only temporarily. But they almost all said that thanks to this experience they no longer felt any fear of death. Some even went as far as to say that they anticipated their death with pleasure. Some spoke of their NDE in a rather odd way, as if they had just returned from a long trip to Japan or some other exotic place. As they came from diverse social contexts and regions across the United States, their interpretations naturally diverged regarding the definition of the famous white light: it was Jesus, or God, or simply Love. But they had all felt an extraordinary and loving energy that had induced in them a degree of happiness that they had trouble describing. They had returned only because they had been forced to.

26

white light

Having caught a glimpse of their deceased loved ones in the nimbus of the loving light, the NDE travellers had only one desire: to remain 'on the other side'. They explained to me that in the preceding days and weeks, these loving friends and family had begun to appear in their dreams, or to pay them friendly, ghostly visits, or to pop up involuntarily in their thoughts. It was as if they wanted to prepare them for the great passage. And when the day came, these deceased grandparents, parents, siblings or spouses had been there, at the end of the tunnel, to welcome them. My patients had been so glad to see them again! But something had told them, 'You're not ready, you have to return to Earth.' And they had woken in their hospital beds with the terrible impression that they had been expelled from Paradise.

Although I was astonished – particularly in the beginning – by these accounts from beyond, I certainly didn't think these patients were crazy. In psychiatry, the notion of insanity is quite precise. It refers to beliefs and behaviour that 1) are not necessary to the person's functioning and 2) will harm the patient. So it's not enough for someone to exhibit unusual beliefs and behaviours to qualify as 'mad'. He or she could just be someone who is out of sync with the era – an eccentric, an artist, et cetera – or someone who is ahead of his or her time – a visionary.

Let's take the case of Jesus or St Paul, Mohammed, or any number of other prophets. A narrow-minded psychiatrist might state that Jesus was a schizophrenic, because he had visions and heard voices; or that he was bipolar, or manic-depressive, because he alternated between episodes of exaltation and periods of depression. Does this mean that Jesus was psychotic? The question seems all the more pertinent because his ideas and actions brought him to a rather undesirable end – which corresponds to the second criterion defining insanity.

In my humble opinion, it is better to renounce these narrow and reductive notions, and see in Jesus a great mind and spirit who was ahead of his time, and perhaps of all time. As for people who say they have 'travelled beyond death', they sometimes return with beliefs that make them stronger. Of course, we shouldn't believe in nonsense just because it makes us feel stronger. But no longer to be terrified of death is nonetheless a wonderful gift! These experiences deserve to be studied if only for the reassurance they could offer. And incidentally, for a scientist they constitute the only available data regarding a state of being that is as important as it is difficult to classify.

On a more modest, personal level, I can say that at the uncomfortable stage at which I find myself today, these accounts are more precious than ever. I accept their inevitable mysterious or 'mystical' dimension, though I can't find in it any argument in favour of one religious dogma or another.

Above all, what I find so satisfying about these beliefs is that they offer me a vision of death which is compatible with my deep and eternal faith in relationships. To be connected to people has always been of central importance to my personal wellbeing. When, at times, I have felt less connected, even if only fleetingly, I have rapidly sunk into sadness and felt my vital energy evaporate. If death is understood to be the cut-off point of all relationships, it becomes, for me, a nightmarish vision: in losing life, I will lose all ties with this source of spiritual nourishment and find myself condemned to absolute solitude. Obviously I realize that dead people aren't supposed to feel anything. But the idea of a dark wasteland deprived of love is chilling.

On the other hand, the prospect of joining the entire community of human and animal souls in a universe that is bathed in light, connectedness and love fills me with joy. Nothing proves that NDE visions actually reflect any kind of reality. It's quite possible that they are no more than the hallucinated product of a handful of neurones misfiring due to a cocktail of chemicals. But from my vantage point today, I'd rather imagine that my death will resemble the famous tunnel leading me to a white light. It would be lovely to be welcomed by the luminous waves of love, and by all the people whom I've loved so much and who died before me: my father, my grandmother, and my beloved grandfather.

27

on love

Since my left arm and leg have become paralysed, and my symptoms show no signs of receding, I've been thinking that this cancer could suddenly accelerate at any moment. So the time has come to take stock of my life. What have I done that has been good and what have I done that has been not so good? Where have I succeeded and where have I fallen short?

On balance I would say that the area I've succeeded the least is in my love life. For mysterious reasons, I haven't managed to love women as I would have liked to. Too often it was as if I remained on the surface of things. Not all the time, but that's one of my greatest regrets.

When I was young, my head was crammed with very misguided ideas on the subject. Love was something that men forced on women because women were by nature reluctant; the only way to go about getting a woman to love you was to subjugate her. A love story was first and foremost a conquest, and then it was the story of an occupation, a pure power struggle, in which the man had every reason to seek and maintain a dominant position. There could be no question of the man relaxing his grip, even after the woman surrendered. As his control was not legitimate, he needed constantly to guard his conquest and keep her subservient to prevent her from rebelling. At the time, it was impossible for me to imagine a harmonious relationship, a bond based on give and take, or any sort of equality between the partners.

I'm still wondering where on earth I picked up these dumb ideas that wrecked all my romantic relationships until I was into my thirties. With my head full of this imperialist concept of love, I tried with all my might to behave like an occupying power. My quest for romance was basically just the search for a domain to conquer. The result: I loved – sometimes madly – but I was not loved back. Or, more precisely, when I was loved (because it did happen occasionally), I didn't allow myself to feel loved, because if I did, then I would have to put down my weapons and accept that I was no longer master of the situation.

My love life during this time when I was at my most imbecilic left me feeling terribly frustrated. For example, I was convinced that women are wired in such a way that they're not at all interested in physical love. But it wasn't only sex: in reality they weren't interested in anything. I thought that they didn't really care that much about going walking, or watching a movie, or eating in a fun restaurant. Whereas I, on the other hand, loved nothing more than a romantic evening out, a dinner for two.

Of course, I did meet women who were delighted to share these things with me, and even wanted to make love with me. But I kept my imperialist cap firmly on. I wasn't going to let myself be swayed or influenced.

How sad that I wasted so much time and so many opportunities to be happy! Twenty years later, there's a trace of this attitude left: my wife often complains that I don't know how to let myself be loved. Happily, I finally got rid of these grotesque ideas. When I was about thirty I made a quantum leap that projected me light-years forward, into an enchanted universe in which women were gifted with intelligence and could share a whole feast of common interests with me. I stopped evaluating the woman I loved against an ideal model she could never match. I understood that in love, as in every other endeavour, the best is the enemy of the good, and the search for perfection is futile.

I was finally able to experience real love, with women who were, on every level, my equal. I learned there was much more pleasure in giving and receiving than in dominating or imposing myself on someone by seduction. In short, I became someone who was more or less all right to hang out with, even if I do still sometimes feel that, in love, I'm lost in uncharted territory, where I have few landmarks and where I'm not always certain how to read the signs.

The intellectual understanding of the general principles of what a more authentic relationship can be brought me an unexpected reward: bizarrely, the spirit of equality within my romantic relationships also spread to my relationships with my patients. I began developing a bond with them, not of love exactly, but of affection that was founded on respect. What an amazing discovery for the rather arrogant young doctor I was! I no longer needed to force myself into a position of control or domination. The relationship could be a two-way process, and I could be enriched by my patients' humanity.

This transformation occurred at the same time that I learned I had cancer, alongside the emotional turmoil that my diagnosis provoked. The realization that I was fragile, mortal, ailing and frightened opened my eyes to the infinite treasures of living and loving. My priorities were thrown upside down, my emotional outlook changed, and the truth is that I felt far happier than I did before – which is surprising.

I also went through a kind of spiritual rebirth. I had been a typical scientist – rational, atheist – and now I found myself in a 'state of grace'. The experience brought me closer to God; and this had become so important for me that when I meditated I found myself trying to speak to God, to communicate with Him. I asked Him to keep me in this extraordinary state of openness and happiness. I thanked Him for the grace that my illness had bestowed upon me, and I promised Him that I would use this light to help others as much as I could.

I experienced this newly incandescent state of being, and then, inexplicably, I lost it. Later, the mystics with whom I discussed it told me that it's a relatively common phenomenon: you find 'grace', and then you lose it. Some people devote the rest of their lives to trying to recapture it.

I'm happy to have lived through such a moment, even if only briefly. When I think of the way in which my life has been transformed, I hope everyone might one day enjoy this experience – preferably without first having to undergo brain surgery. It's essentially the goal of psychotherapy, and it's what psychotherapy achieves when it's 'successful'. People who have been helped by methods such as EMDR, behavioural and cognitive therapies or meditation undergo something like this blossoming, this rebirth. I'm convinced that we can also achieve this goal if we adopt a lifestyle that's respectful of global ecology (the network of nature and of human relationships). This is the lifestyle I call 'anticancer'. I expressed this desire at the end of my book: if we avoid everything that damages life, and instead encourage and promote everything that nourishes it, we can develop the wonderful resources that are hidden within us. It will give us a new perspective on the world around us: on nature, on our children, on our work. We will discover our ability to give with generosity and receive with gratitude. All this is vitally important, and it is not limited to people with cancer.

28

vital interactions

Two decades ago, when I was a researcher in neuroscience, I spent a lot of time looking at the structure of neurones. I was struck by the fact that the vast and fascinating network of connections that we call the brain is composed of cells which, looked at individually, are neither very intelligent nor particularly competent. But as soon as they interact they give rise to the most brilliant mental faculties: phenomena such as perception, intelligence, creativity, memory and so on. We term these phenomena 'emergent' because they exceed to an infinite degree the capacities of the entities from which they arise; they result, in fact, from the actions and return actions that are constantly operating between them.

Later, I understood that the entire body also functions on this network model. The liver interacts constantly with the kidneys, which interact with blood pressure, blood quality, urine production, hormones and so on. Like the neurone systems, the organism also produces emergent properties. And just as for the brain, these properties constitute a kind of intelligence, the 'intelligence of the body' which we more often refer to as 'health'.

For what is health, if not the result of the harmonious and balanced performance of all the systems that together make up the body? When this performance goes awry, it is pointless to dwell only on the ailing organ – the liver, blood, heart or whatever. Instead, we must seek to restore the equilibrium of the whole.

The wisdom of ancestral medical traditions, such as Ayurvedic, Chinese, or Tibetan medicine, is based on the understanding that caring for the sick means re-establishing equilibrium within the body, not just focusing on a specific problem. It is this holistic philosophy that inspired me to create in Pittsburgh one of the first centres for integrative medicine, where patients are offered both conventional and alternative treatments. I'm convinced that the ancient traditions have a lot to teach us. It would be extremely useful to study them, select a few, and integrate some of their practices into our repertoire of care.

Adopting a more systemic point of view within Western medical practice would in itself represent a step forward. For example, faced with a painful joint, we should attempt to care not for that particular joint, but for the more global problem of arthritis that affects the whole organism. Of course, it is sometimes necessary to deal with a specific problem, such as a failing appendix that is endangering the entire body. This is the enormous success of modern medicine, which I'm the first to applaud: to have found effective methods to manage crisis situations such as heart attacks or pneumonia, for example. But we can neither understand nor preserve health if we narrow our intervention to isolated problems. Health can be properly addressed only on the larger scale of the entire organism – or even on the scale of nature, as everything is so interconnected.

I'm very happy to see the doctors with whom I have the most dealings at the moment – oncologists – becoming receptive to a more systemic vision of their profession. They have stopped focusing exclusively on the tumour and are now progressively integrating the richer notion of 'the terrain'. They have begun to explore nutrition, physical activity, psychological dimensions and more. There's nothing mystical or esoteric about this attitude, it is simply holistic.

To take the classic example of antibiotics that kill all bacteria, good as well as bad: we are aware that these medications upset the intestinal flora and cause diarrhoea. A holistic vision would consist of prescribing, alongside such antibiotics, bacteria to preserve the intestinal flora; and fortunately this is what many physicians are now doing. This trend will spread, little by little, into chemotherapy, radiotherapy and even surgery. A whole series of preparatory measures already exists to lessen bleeding, minimize post-operative pain, and so on. It is unthinkable not to put them into practice in hospitals.

More generally, I'm convinced that medicine has reached the limits of a model based on seeking out a 'miracle drug'. There are indeed a few diseases we can deal with adequately via a single medication: insulin for diabetes, for example. It's a remarkable treatment that certainly should not be abandoned. But it's difficult to see how we could find one single drug to treat illnesses that are inherently systemic, such as obesity, cancer or high blood pressure. We can try to reduce blood pressure through medication, but the underlying problem won't be resolved this way. And we will not be able to find the pharmaceutical molecule that conquers coronary artery disease, because this syndrome affects all the arteries: no medication can clean up all of them. However, it's been proven that thirty minutes on a stationary bike five times a week is more effective against heart disease than inserting a stent.

In reality, both types of approach are useful and – this is my profound belief – they are perfectly complementary. Someone who has just had a heart attack shouldn't be saddling up his bike straight away. He needs a stent, immediately, and that will save his life. But in the months and years that follow, he would be well advised to do some cycling, or else the stent will clog up again.

The major obstacle to the development of integrative medicine is that it doesn't generate opportunities to make lots of money. When a pharmaceutical laboratory discovers a medication or perfects a new stent, it hits the jackpot: the patent will be incredibly lucrative. But if one were to discover that by massaging a certain acupuncture point the need for anti-inflammatory medication could be reduced by 30 per cent, this action couldn't be patented and would not create an industry. Only health-insurance systems could benefit from it – although, for reasons that are difficult to understand, they hardly ever do.

My American friends envy the European system of health insurance. They imagine that, for economic reasons, it is receptive to more intelligent approaches to health. I used to agree. I used to think the French social-welfare system would be interested in the rigorous studies that establish the effects of acupuncture, or yoga, on certain diseases. There is evidence, for example, that treating two acupuncture points reduces by 60 per cent the need for morphine after an operation. Having often taken care of older people following surgery, it is clear to me how useful it would be to reduce these doses, because morphine makes the elderly confused and leads to nightmares and hallucinations. They fall out of their beds at night and break their legs; they often end up dying in hospital. Whether you look at it from a human, medical or economic perspective, the only rational thing to do is to prescribe acupuncture. Tragically, this doesn't happen. Why not? The only explanation I've been able to come up with is that it's because no one earns any money from it.

I was actually naive enough to suggest to the directors of the French health-insurance system that a small fraction of their budget should be earmarked for exploring new techniques that might lead to significant savings. I was amazed. The administrators I met – all intelligent and conscientious people – were so obsessed with the need to cut spending that they seemed unable to grasp the point of investing a minimal sum in order to reap long-term savings.

The way we approach healthcare is a reflection of a whole series of burning questions that define our era. This problem has been well put by my friend Michael Lerner: 'Healthy people cannot exist on a sick planet.' This is where health becomes a part of our global ecology. There's even a new discipline that has emerged at the interface of these different fields: *eco-medicine*, which was founded at a worldwide level by Lerner. It looks at public health problems linked with mobile phone technology, pesticides and fertilizers, radiation (which is more relevant than ever in the aftermath of the Fukushima Daiichi event in Japan), drinking water and the food industry.

An unexpected and extremely encouraging movement has sprung up in the food industry that questions the old ways of looking at these problems. I'm thinking of the role played in recent years by consumer groups, and the realization that there is food being sold to us that actually poisons us. Incidentally, it is also a good example of the way networks can operate: consumers' interest sparks that of the media, which leads in turn to an even greater surge of public interest. As a result, there are many supermarket chains that have been obliged to listen to their customers, and make available bigger ranges of organic food and natural products.

The example is inspiring – it gives us the hope of changing our entire agricultural system from the bottom up. More and more farmers realize that they need to convert to organic methods; not just for the good of their soil, or their own health, but also for economic reasons, because organic produce will enable them to increase their revenue. It's about time! Take grapevines, for instance: because of the chemicals used to fight phylloxera, wine contains one thousand times the dose of pesticide that is tolerated in drinking water. Perhaps this makes sense at an industrial level, but when it comes to public health, it's completely insane. And yet there are solutions. Organic wine exists, and I bet that wine-lovers will not put up for much longer with the prospect of absorbing a soup of pesticides every time they feel like sipping a glass of fine wine.

The way we treat the animals we eat is both outrageous and appalling. Once I learned how battery hens are treated, for example, I could no longer eat them. A huge sea-change is underway in people's attitudes on this point, and I think the food industry will rapidly need to overhaul a system that is destructive not only to the environment but also to public health.

The most egregious example is that of pesticides and fertilizers. Their use on a massive scale leads to the destruction of the soil and the contamination of our food. Washed away by rain, they go on to pollute rivers and seas, leading to dangerous phenomena such as algae blooms and sex changes in certain amphibians and fish. When these fish end up on our plates, they contribute to drastically increased rates of cancer.

Ecology teaches us that every form of life is the expression of communication and exchange within a network. The earth itself functions as a whole, where almost everything interacts all the time. Here too, these interactions generate emergent properties that constitute the 'intelligence of the Earth'. It's this intelligence that we sabotage when we deliberately violate the Earth's natural balance. Fortunately, we've become aware of this; as far as I am concerned, our understanding of how the mechanisms of these networks function constitutes our major progress of the past thirty or forty years.

A report commissioned by the French research agency INSERM (National Institute of Health and Medical Research) has recognized that environmental factors are of considerable significance in the current epidemic of cancer. These factors range from atmospheric pollution to radiation, via the infinite range of chemical molecules that are present in our everyday life. We need to attack the root of the problem by putting an end to the poisoning of our environment and reforming the food industry. Instead, 97 per cent of our research effort is oriented towards methods of treatment and detection of cancer. I'm a firm believer that our health is intrinsically linked to the health of our environment. Heal our planet and we will heal ourselves.

29

when the wind blows

As I draw up this balance sheet of my life, I would gladly put my professional activity in the positive column. I think I've worked hard; perhaps too hard, given the consequences, but I don't regret having thrown myself wholeheartedly into my work. I've learned some fascinating things, which I've been happy to put to the service of the greater good. I feel I've been useful, and this gives a great deal of meaning to my life as I look back on it.

My oncologist tells me that patients come to see him almost every day with a copy of *Anticancer* under their arm. They talk about what they can do to play an active role in the fight against their tumour. These patients, who were previously wallowing in discouragement, suddenly begin telling him, 'I realize there are things that I can do to help *you* help *me*.' Their behaviour changes: they adhere to treatment protocols with much more discipline, courage and willpower. My oncologist is delighted to see these patients escape from the grip of depression, which is known to have a negative impact on remission and survival. There are no words to describe the satisfaction I derive from knowing that in some small way I helped give confidence and hope to these patients – my brothers and sisters – in their time of need.

Nothing touches me more than those readers who, when they come to ask me to sign a book or a programme after a lecture, say to me, 'Thanks to you, I regained hope and began to really fight. You've made me understand that I can do something for myself.' Each time, I am moved and filled with gratitude. I feel as though I have given them a precious gift: the realization that we all possess inner strength. When I sign their books, I often write about the strength these readers have within themselves. If they think about that source of strength, they're already halfway to being saved. Even if their tumour doesn't disappear, even if their treatment fails, they will have taken an active part in shaping their fate, and this is perhaps enough to help them to be at peace with themselves.

· According to Marshall Rosenberg, the genius who invented the principle of non-violent communication, the main source of meaning in life is through contributing to the wellbeing of those around us. It's true of all humans, and probably of animals too. We see it, for example, in a professional context. Studies show that what makes people proud of their work isn't so much their salary or their status in the hierarchy; it's the conviction that the products they manufacture, or the services they offer, contribute to the wellbeing of others. This is why some professions have a satisfaction index that is higher than others. And incidentally, this satisfaction isn't just reserved for people who have jobs: all human relationships provide opportunities to contribute to the happiness of other people.

This is particularly true with one's own family. Contributing to the wellbeing of your spouse gives profound pleasure. Contributing to the happiness of your children is pure joy. Nothing can give more meaning to our lives. My children are among my life's most wonderful achievements.

And yet, when I think of Charlie and Anna, who are so young, I am filled with great sadness. I'm constantly talking about 'giving back', but I fear I will not be able to do that for these two wonderful beings who need it the most. I hope, all the same, that I will leave them an image of me that will help them as they grow. I think of the video messages I will record for them with my webcam, and the letters I will write. I will talk to them about my hopes for them, and what I already see in them: the source of their zest for life. I will tell them how sad I am not to be present in their lives, and about my conviction that they have within themselves what they need to grow up in my absence: the memory, even blurred or indirect, that they will keep of me. And, above all, their mother's strength.

But as long as I still have the hope of recovering, I put the project off till later. I'm in no rush. But I keep turning over in my mind the words I will use. When the time comes, I hope I'll be fit enough to record these messages. Perhaps it's a good exercise to do this even when we're in perfect health: to work out what we would say to our children if we knew we were about to die.

With my elder son, Sacha, I'm happy to say I've talked about it openly. The fact that he lives far away has long been a source of suffering for me; when we saw each other at Christmas, I suggested that he and his mother could return to live in France. I told him that I didn't know how much more time I would have and I wanted to spend these few months together. He looked at me and began to cry. 'You know, Dad, it's so hard having a sick father...'

We wept together. It was difficult, yes, but we were able to talk about it. For each of us, that moment was both terribly upsetting and very useful, because it permitted us to express to each other the pain we felt. I know that Sacha is grieving; every time I hear his voice on the phone or see his face on the computer screen, I'm struck by his sadness. But I like to think that these moments of shared emotion will be an important keepsake when he connects with me in his memory.

Sometimes I fantasize that when they grow up, my children will feel protected by a thin enveloping veil, as if a benevolent force were floating around them. As if, on my way out, I had left them something of myself, an immaterial part that cannot be seen, heard, or touched, but which can be felt. A force of unconditional love that is always ready to support them, lead them, encourage them.

Sometimes I even imagine that this part of me has the power of consciousness, and that it will somehow succeed in supporting those I love in their mourning. It would be wonderful to be able to instil in my children the strength, courage and desire to contribute to the greater good when they grow up. Then I will be able to pass over completely to 'the other side', with my heart at peace.

I know that my grandparents and my father continue to live in me. It's a well-known psychological truth: when we lose someone close to us, a person whom we've loved, something of what they have bestowed on us continues to live within us and inspire us. Our dead live in our hearts. It's the most comforting form of immortality, and the one that means the most to me.

There's a line I love from a letter that a soldier wrote to his wife when he was leaving to fight in the American Civil War. There wasn't much chance that he'd come home alive. If he didn't, he wrote, he hoped that every time she felt a breeze on her face, she would know he was there.

I would like to share that image, that intuition, with my wife and children, so that when they feel the gentle caress of the wind on their faces, they can say, 'Hey, it's Dad, come back to kiss me.'

afterword

My brother David died just eight weeks after completing this book. The way in which he approached his death is a lesson for life.

Thirteen months elapsed between the diagnosis of his tumour and his passing on 24 July 2011. Throughout, David fought the disease like a bull in an arena: with as much courage as lucidity about his odds of winning the battle – which he knew to be statistically nill – and with as much will to live as humility in the face of his prognosis.

When the tumour came back after months of high-tech procedures and painful follow-up treatments, he knew – we all knew – that he had very little time left. So he embraced life's ultimate trial, that of dying well. He viewed it as his final challenge, so as to feel empowered rather than helpless. He chose to fully exploit the possibilities offered by this strange period of life that he knew to be his last.

As the cancer continued to grow in his brain, it invaded his motor cortex, paralysing his limbs one after the other, confusing his eyesight, shutting his voice down to a faint whisper, and reducing his ability to concentrate to fewer and fewer hours per day. David dedicated all his remaining physical and mental strength to the writing of this book, in the hope that his own experience could help others.

That this book exists at all is a miracle. It was snatched just in time from the jaws of his disease. It is David's most personal book and he was deeply moved by his readers' enthusiasm for it. With his strength dwindling, just days before he died, he held up the French bestseller list to his eyes, to see his book at the top. It gave him the feeling of having defied the cancer in a most meaningful way. He had not allowed it to get in the way of his being useful, of his helping alleviate other people's suffering.

Until the end, David remained a doctor at heart, a healer.

Those of us who had the privilege of taking care of him, of accompanying him in his ordeal, often had the feeling that it was he who was taking care of us. He would meet our clumsiness with limitless patience; he would dissipate with a grateful gaze any embarrassment caused by his extreme physical dependence on us. He took care of our souls.

I remember how, a few days before the end, he lay on his hospital bed, unable to speak and almost entirely paralysed. At this stage of the agony, his means of communication were reduced to some movements of his right hand and the brows above his deep blue eyes. As I covered his hand with mine, in an attempt to reassure him and give him some of my strength, I was surprised when, a moment later, looking straight up at me, he freed himself to cover my hand with his. I understood then that he wanted to reassure *me* that everything would be all right!

At one point in this book, David wonders candidly about his store of courage and asks us to forgive him should he tremble at the edge of death.

You should know that he never trembled. He departed peacefully, listening to the playlist he had assembled for this purpose; he stepped over to the other side while Daniel Barenboim played the second movement of Mozart's 23rd piano concerto.

David was not afraid of death. He believed it would transport him to a kingdom of love, through the famous tunnel of light so often described by those who have had a near-death experience.

May it be so, my brother.

For your part, you gave us an extraordinary example of what we might call a 'successful death experience'. A precious parting gift to hold in our hearts, so that, from time to time, we can draw from it some of the strength necessary to confront life.

Emile Servan-Schreiber
Paris, 27 July 2011

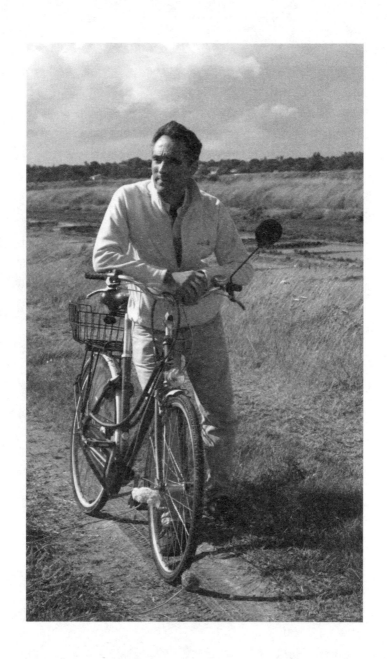